a positive life

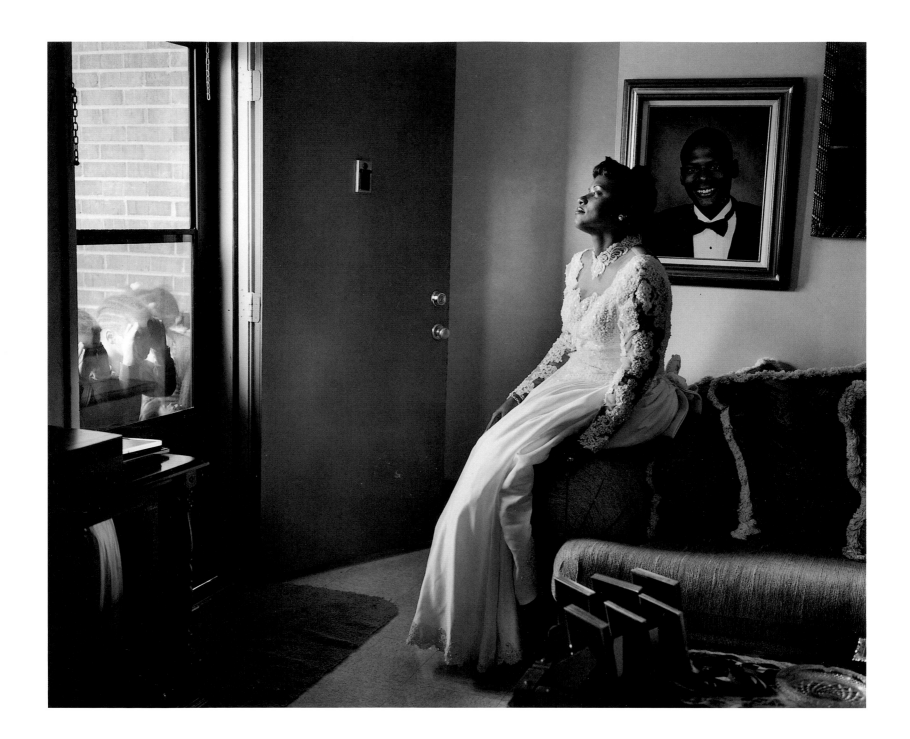

a positive life

Portraits of Women
Living with HIV

Interviews by River Huston • Photographs by Mary Berridge

RUNNING PRESS
PHILADELPHIA · LONDON

Text © 1997 by River Huston
Photographs © 1997 by Mary Berridge
All rights reserved under the Pan-American and International Copyright Conventions
Printed in China

Library of Congress Cataloging-in-Publication Number 96-72481

ISBN 0-7624-0198-2 hardcover
ISBN 0-7624-0244-X paperback

Designed by Maria Taffera Lewis
Edited by Greg Jones
Typography: Goudy Old Style

This book may be ordered by mail from the publisher.
Please include $2.50 for postage and handling.
But try your bookstore first!

Running Press Book Publishers
125 South Twenty-second Street
Philadelphia, Pennsylvania 19103-4399

This book is dedicated to all women living with HIV.

—*R. H. and M. B.*

contents

acknowledgments

We would like to thank all the women who participated in this project and all the women who gave of their time and their heart but were not included in this book. A special thanks to the people who helped us find women to photograph, in particular: Juanita Williams in Georgia, Nancy MacNeil and all the women at Women Alive in Los Angeles, Sandy Luna and Anna Heeks in San Francisco, and a special thanks to Andrea and Ben Acosta for their generous hospitality.

This project was funded in part by generous grants from the Center for Documentary Studies at Duke University; the Maine Photographic Workshops; and the New York Foundation for the Arts. Thank-you, Running Press, for believing in our project.

I give a special thanks to Dawn Averitt for starting the Women's Information Service and Exchange (WISE) in Atlanta, and to Rebecca Denison for creating Women Organized to Respond to Life-threatening Diseases (WORLD)— both of these women have been a powerful example to many women living with HIV/AIDS. Thank you to Misha Cohen, Michelle Lopez, Marlena Diaz, Marion Banzhaf, Abigail Surasky, Lark Lands, Jill Makin, Phyillipa Lawson, Julie Davids, Pam Ladds, Paula Toyton, Anna Forbes, and Irene Snow for all their dedication and effort in helping affected women with treatment and healing, both social and emotional.

I would also like to thank the healers who have helped to keep me well—Dr. Rosemary Harris, Dr. Susan Weir, Dr. Patricia Erceg, Bert Rinkel, and Sherri Simon. A grateful thanks to Vanessa Vandergrift for keeping my world straight while I was on the road. My deepest thanks to Rick Poverny-Benjerman for sharing his love, insights, and support. Abba Rolland for being a dedicated friend. Geoffrey Teague for his loving encouragement. And lastly, to my sweet little Yorkshire "terrorist," Buddy.

RH

I would like to thank the following people for their input and encouragement: Richard Benson, Jennie Dunham, Alex Harris, Geoffrey Hutchinson, Susan Kismaric, Laura Letinsky, Tanya Marcuse, Tod Papageorge, Evie Papastephanou, Michael Spano, and Eric Weeks. Also, I would like to give a special thanks to Jennette Williams for her friendship and for going over every single contact sheet for this project. Finally, I would like to thank my parents for their understanding and support, and my fiance, Clark Troy, for his wise advice, sympathetic ear, and unceasing editorial vigilance.

MB

preface

In 1993, I started a job interviewing mothers with AIDS and their teen-age children for psychological research studies. The job took me all around the New York area, on subways and buses, to the most remote corners of the boroughs, and I entered the homes of countless families. I would sit with these women and barrage them with a litany of dry and invasive questions: "How many times would you say you drank alcoholic beverages in the past three months?" "Do you have enough money every day to eat three well-balanced meals?" "How many times have you had sex in the last three months?" I asked the teenagers a similar list of questions, and thus I produced the clinical data necessary for the quantitative study.

At the same time it struck me that the actual lives of these HIV-positive women were all but invisible. One could read in the paper that women, and in particular lower-income women, were the fastest growing segment of the HIV-infected community—but beyond that they were drastically underrepresented in both the mass media and the arts. And here these women were before me, struggling with their illness, working, raising children, taking care of their homes, and coping with a sense of vulnerability and uncertainty unknown to most of us.

I had recently completed a series of photographs of teen mothers, and I wasn't really sure what I wanted to photograph next. But meeting these women, seeing what their lives were like, and talking to them put an end to my confusion. At first it was difficult finding women to photograph. Why would anyone want to have her picture taken if going public would expose her to stigmatization and prejudice? I contacted support groups and social-service agencies; I placed ads in newsletters. Slowly, women began to call me back, and I hauled my camera and tripod onto the same subways and buses I had ridden for my interviewing job, only this time I was not trying to reduce their individual experiences to a set of numbers.

About a year after I began working on this project, a woman from New Hope, Pennsylvania, answered one of my ads, so I boarded a train and went out to photograph her. She immediately impressed me with her openness and ribald sense of humor. She even suggested that we do some nudes. On top of this, she patiently answered my prying and somewhat naive questions (for instance: "Do you and your boyfriend have sex?"). I had been looking for a writer to record the stories of the women I was photographing and I wanted that person to be involved in the community of HIV-positive women. Well, she was a writer and she was definitely involved. This woman was River Huston.

When I was in training for my interviewing job it was emphasized that I should be "objective" and nonjudgemental so as not to prejudice the "data." When I had to ask such questions as "Have you thought about who will take care of your children when you die?" for example, I never knew how to pose them "objectively." Even if it was designed to elicit a simple yes or no answer, the question itself bore so much emotional weight as to render such an answer almost meaningless.

My photographs are not objective. They are very much my own vision of what makes my subjects' lives compelling. At the same time, I have tried to present the women I have photographed as honestly as I could—in their own environments—so that the specificity of their lives would be both palpable and realized.

Mary Berridge

introduction

In terms of both length and number of interviews, this book is directly influenced by the perception of HIV disease in the popular imagination. Fear of losing jobs and insurance benefits, fear of losing the love of family members and friends, and especially fear of the discrimination their children would face if their stories became public kept many of the women I interviewed from allowing their words to be published in this volume. Their fear is not to be taken lightly, as any woman, man, or child living with HIV disease well knows. Between the lines, as it were, these women are nevertheless still given voice here: together they whisper that anonymity remains a necessary strategy to resist some of the nastier, more pernicious cultural sanctions and reactions associated with HIV disease. May there be another day, another book, another wholly accepting public forum in which these women can tell their stories without fear.

What's missing from this book, however, is more than compensated by what remains. The bravery, courage, and commitment of the women you will meet in these pages is both representative and exemplary. Listening, transcribing, asking questions—the whole interview process always had me on the verge of tears. Hearing these stories at once took its toll and kept me going. It meant defying doctors' orders to stay in bed; listening and writing through my own bout with pneumonia; and painstakingly transcribing interviews during long stretches on the road while someone else was thankfully doing the driving. All the while, I kept reminding myself how important these words, voices, and women were, and how what might be "bad for you" (in terms of health) in another way is good for the soul.

Even though I have become immune to the tragedy of my own story, I cannot help being affected by the sadness, power, and courage of what I have heard over the last three years while we have been working on this book. The stories these women have told me are infectious. Certain words and phrases reverberate, returning to me at the most ordinary moments. I am making breakfast or walking the dog and remember Laurie's husband, Steve, saying to someone who has asked if he isn't afraid of losing his wife: "Our forever is not like your forever."

As a woman living with HIV disease myself, I have often been the one interviewed; the one answering the questions. Like many of the women in this book I have been frequently misquoted, misunderstood, or censored beyond all recognition. Such experiences dictated the method of this book so that the voices of these women would be honored almost as if I was an oral ethnographer instead of an interviewer or editor. Quite simply, I would let them tell their stories, transcribe them, read them back, and pay the phone bills later.

I believe in the truth of these voices, and trust they have something to teach us about what it is like to be a woman living in the late-twentieth century with a disease that provokes anger, hatred, and denial, yet somehow inspires in us equal measures of compassion, faith, and humanity. This book sets out to document such extremes in the hope of moving all of us towards a response to this epidemic that we can look back on as honorable.

lery espinosa

27, diagnosed HIV-positive in 1994, infected through sex

Physically, I feel fine. Emotionally it's a burden that I have to carry every day. I got tested because I knew that I had been at risk. I just needed to make sure I was okay. I didn't really think that I would actually test positive. I went to my private doctor and asked for an HIV test. He told me that I wasn't really at risk and I didn't need to take this test. I insisted on it, and finally he agreed. Two weeks later they called me from the doctor's office. I really didn't pay that much attention because I was sure that it was negative. When I realized it was the doctor that kept calling me, I went in right away.

First he told me that my iron levels were low. Then he said, 'Lery, unfortunately the other test came back positive, the test for the HIV.' I thought, 'Oh my God! I can't believe it!' I started crying. He tried to comfort me. He told me that there was a lot of trial medicine available now. He told me

not to kiss my kids. I was just so worried about my kids. I was totally ignorant about the subject. I thought I was going to die right away or in the next six months. I couldn't stop crying for about two and a half hours. Then I tried to go home and act like nothing had happened.

When I got home, my mom saw my face and realized that I had been crying. I made up a story about having a fight with my husband. I made up my mind not to tell anyone about it, even my husband. But that night my husband came home from school and he told me about this essay that he had written. It was about me. How important I was in his life. I broke down and started crying. Finally I told him. He hugged me and said, 'Oh honey,' and he started crying. He didn't know what to say. That night I cried myself to sleep.

I also told my sister, and she made me tell my father and

2

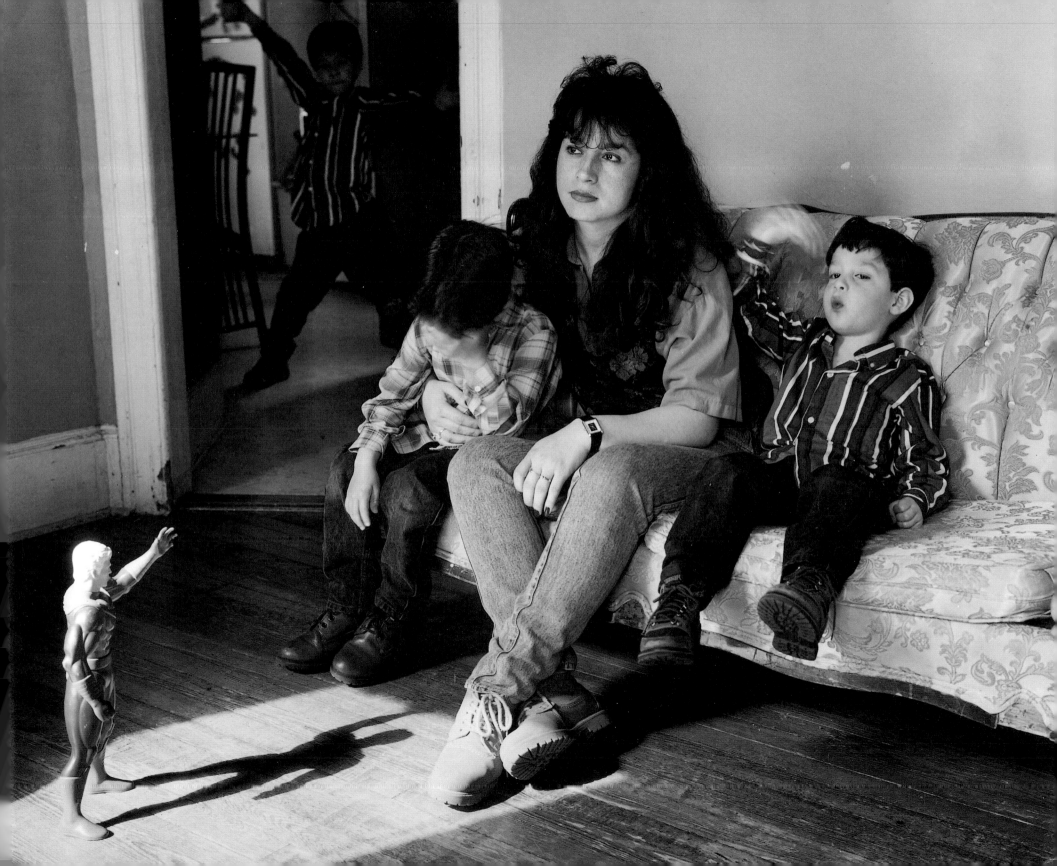

my mother. They started looking for support groups for all of us. They found a support group for me. In the group they talked about how important it was to get rid of all the stress in my life. I knew what that meant for me.

Before this had happened, my husband and I had been having problems. We had been separated for a while and just recently had gotten back together. I said, 'It's my life and I really have to make a final decision about this.' I asked him to leave. We used to fight all the time. I had to be on top of him to do everything. We already had three kids—I didn't need a fourth one. He was like a grown-up kid. He has remained a good friend and is very supportive.

My first experience going out with someone after I found out I was positive taught me a lot. I didn't tell the guy I was dating. I didn't feel strong enough to tell him. I was in a stage of denial. We went out for about four months. What woke me up was that I got pregnant. I thought, 'Oh my God, what am I doing?' We always used a condom, but there were a couple of times when it slipped off. I went through the whole process of terminating the pregnancy. I felt I had to tell this guy because I must have put him at risk. I had my sister call him up and tell him. She told him that I just found out that I was HIV-positive. He was very

scared. He went and got tested. It was negative, thank God. I called him three months later and reminded him to get tested again. I don't know if he went. I'm always safe now. I tell before I do anything.

My kids are eight, six, and four—

Jimmy, Nelson, and Manny. They know about HIV. They know that it's a virus. That it comes through your body through sex and IV drug use. That it never leaves. That the doctors have not been able to find the medicine to make it leave your body. That it takes awhile before you get sick, and that people die from AIDS. They don't know that I have it.

In some ways, I think they know. My little one, Manny, he's four and a half. At school he made a poster. Everybody had to do a poster about their mom. He wrote on his poster, 'I wish my mom will never get sick.' I ask myself if they know; can they feel it? My oldest one, Jimmy, gets very worried when I feel sick. Even if it's just a simple headache, he cries. That tells me a lot. I wish I could tell them. I have spoken with their school psychologist and many people who I think have more experience in this kind of thing. They think it's too early to tell them.

My kids know about HIV. They know that it's
a virus. . . . That it never leaves. That people die from AIDS.
. . . They don't know that I have it.

I was once taking an herbal treatment. I had to take it after every meal. The kids would still be eating while I was taking these pills. They would ask me, 'Mom, why do you have to take that?' I would tell them 'I have to take care of you. I go to the gym. I have to go to school. And mommy needs a lot of energy to do all that.' I felt I was lying to them. Here I'm trying to teach them to trust me, and I'm lying to them.

I'm thinking of telling them this summer. They will not have the stress of school, and they can see every day I'm healthy and doing well.

I'm not afraid of dying—I'm more afraid of the physical pain before dying. I guess I try to believe that I'm not going to die from AIDS, but then a lot of fear comes to me about my status. I ask myself, am I really going to die from it or not? You die when it's your time even when you're healthy.

My lifestyle gives me a lot of hope. I exercise. I love dancing. I don't drink or smoke. I am studying International Business at school. I hope to have my own import-export company. I want to try to have my kids' education assured. I don't want them to go through any problems when it comes to higher education. I'm planning to work really hard so they have the money for college when they need it. It's my first priority when it comes to the future.

I'm very close to my family. We all live together—my parents, my sister and her son, my kids and myself. It's a very crowded apartment but it works for now. I feel very supported by my family.

Before I went back to school, I asked my kids if they were willing to make that sacrifice, if they were willing to be a little uncomfortable. If not, we could move to our own apartment and I could work. My oldest said, 'No mommy, you go back to school for two more years, then we can move.' We are very close.

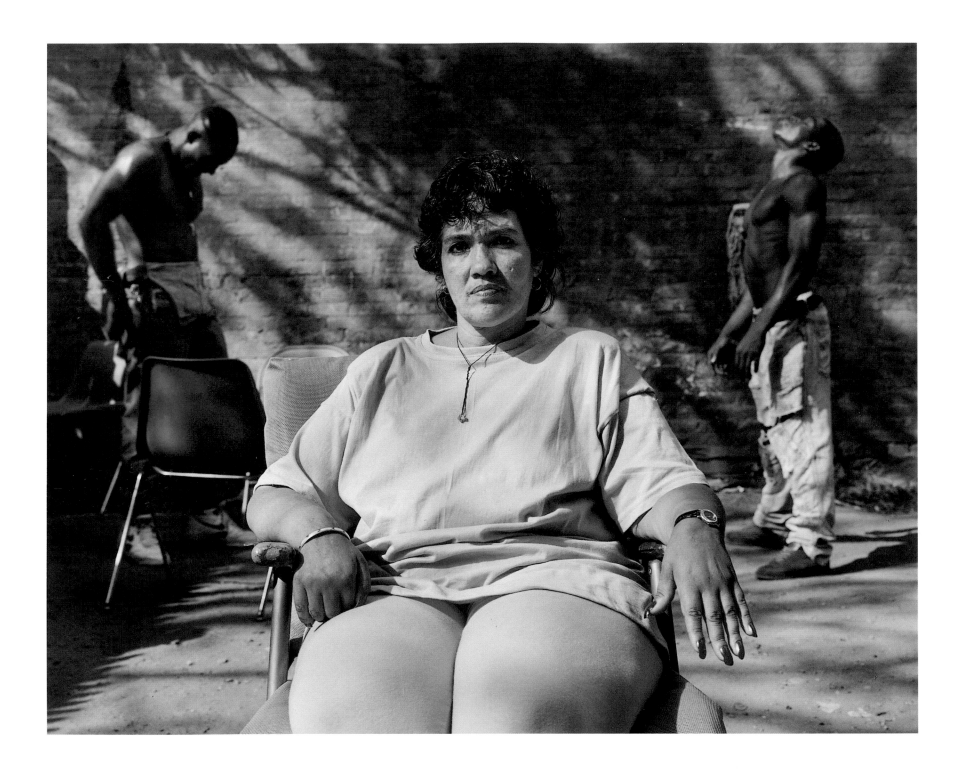

It was the summer of 1985. Someone told me that this health center would pay me twenty dollars to take an HIV test, so I went down there. They gave me some clothes, some stamps for McDonalds, and twenty bucks. They said they would give me another twenty dollars if I came back in two weeks to get my test result. I went back two weeks later. They told me that I was HIV-positive. I was a little upset, but I didn't really know what it meant. They just said I had this HIV virus. There was no real explanation. They told me to go to the Department of Health. I didn't bother going because I wasn't sick. I was just dope sick; other than that I was fine. They never explained nothing like how it was transmitted. I ignored that until 1987.

I was admitted into Lutheran Hospital with endocarditis. The doctor told me about shooting up drugs. He said that was how I got HIV. I was released and went back on the streets. In November I was admitted again for endocarditis. This time I was put in Woodhull Hospital in Brooklyn. I had a very high fever and chronic diarrhea. I had lost a lot of weight. These doctors came in and asked if I wanted to go into a program in Arizona. They would help me get off drugs. They told me that I had to quit sharing needles because I would pick up other diseases. They never asked about my sex life. On the street, HIV was called 'the gay plague.' I was a heterosexual but worked as a prostitute. I didn't know if some of my customers were gay. I really didn't understand it at all. I never got to go to Arizona. I went back on the streets.

In January 1988, I was raped and shot three times while I was working as a prostitute. After that I became a lookout for the drug dealers. I was arrested and I was sent upstate to

lucy rivera

43, HIV-positive since 1985, infected through IV drugs

Albion Correctional Facility. I was there two years. Then I went down state to Taconic Correctional Facility. I was discharged after a few months. While I was up at Albion I learned about unsafe sex and sharing needles. They taught us about the progressions of AIDS. When I was released, I violated my parole by changing my address. I was back on the streets and homeless.

I eventually ended up at Rikers in the Steps program. It was a self-taught empowerment program for people from Rikers. At my graduation I heard this woman, Phyllis Anderson, speak. She stood up and said that she was HIV-positive. She had been an addict and an inmate. Now she was the coordinator at Stand-Up Harlem. She said she has a number and it's not an inmate number! It's her social security number and a telephone number. I was really impressed with her. I liked how she had changed her life. I wanted to change my life. I didn't want to spend the rest of my life in jails, being an addict, being a loser. I went to Stand-Up Harlem and stayed

there. They talked to me about self-esteem and doing positive things for myself. I went to Narcotics Anonymous and Alcoholics Anonymous.

I started to speak around the community. I'm a community activist now. I try to help other people who are addicts and HIV-positive. I try to help people who are still in prison so when they get out they will know where to get help. I'm a certified alcohol counselor and a pre- and post-HIV-test counselor.

When I was using, I was very suicidal. Now I just want to live. I didn't understand anything about love then. I had no one to love me. I was fourteen when I had my son and fifteen when I had my daughter. I never had anyone ever being concerned about me. Never had anyone to nurture me. I remember many times I was hungry and there was no food. There were times I was lonely and crying; I had no one to console me.

Now I have my family. I have a two-bedroom apartment. I volunteer at Stand-Up Harlem. I can be a productive part of society. My own goal is to stop getting Supplemental

Social Security. I want to be able to take care of myself and my family.

I have my three children living with me now. They were all put in foster care when they were little. They're teenagers now. I talk to them about my life as an addict. I also talk to them about safe sex. It's good to be reunited with them. They had the same resentment that I had against my parents: basically, not being there when they were little. Now they have a counselor at Stand-Up Harlem to help them deal with their resentments. Both girls and my boy have been tested for HIV. I think that they will be safe—especially my son, Francisco.

He once had unprotected sex with a woman who turned out to be HIV-positive. After that he took the test, and it was negative. I think that experience really affected him. Since then, he says that he is always safe.

I try to take good care of myself by getting regular check-ups, exercising, and nurturing myself. I know I could never do any of that if I was still using drugs.

I see people go in and out of Stand-Up Harlem. They go back on the streets and use. Every time they come back, they're sicker and sicker. I know that people who go back on drugs die quicker. At Stand-Up Harlem, 12 people died in 1995. In 1996, six people have already died. All of them went back out and used drugs.

Physically, there is a lot going on. I have a sleeping disorder and peripheral neuropathy. My T-cells are 505. They went up from 168. I have been diagnosed with AIDS because I have had chronic and recurrent fevers, diarrhea, and bronchial asthma. I had to have a biopsy recently. I had a lot of bumps under my skin. They didn't know what it was and they have never seen it before. It's only on the areas where I used to shoot up. These bumps are very tender and bluish purple.

In general I feel okay, but it's hard for me to walk. I'm tired a lot. When I came out of jail I weighed 155 pounds; now I'm 260. I took a gland treatment thinking it was my glands. I'm like a box of surprises. It's either herpes, diarrhea, these strange bumps, or my neuropathy. It seems it's always something!

When I visit the hospital and I see these people hooked up to all these tubes, I know I don't want to go through that kind of prolonged pain. I ask God, please let me go in my sleep. I'm really scared. I don't want to go through any more pain. I don't want my family to have to suffer emotional pain.

I'm only 43. I'm not ready to die. I want to see sixty—at least sixty.

We had just moved down to Florida. I wasn't feeling very well and we didn't know any doctors down there. We went to a doctor who turned out to be an Infectious Disease Physician. He tested me for everything. It took about a month to find out what the problem was.

I was in a little room lying on the exam table when the doctor walked in. He looks at me and says, 'I looked at your test, and you're HIV-positive.' He just said it point blank that I was HIV-positive. He never asked my consent to take an HIV test. When he told me, I just blanked out. I felt like I was falling. I had come alone. He asked if I thought I would be able to sleep that night, and he gave me a prescription for Demerol. He did not explain anything to me. He didn't direct me, educate, or help me find out where I could get any support. He was very detached.

I went home and told my husband, Al. Since they found it in me first, he thought it was all my fault and started accusing me of all kinds of things. He was very angry and not supportive or caring about my feelings at all. We had been together seven years. He went to get tested the following week and his test came back positive. Then he really hit the roof. We discussed it in very loud terms. I told him it could've been him giving it to me because it's easier to give to a woman.

HIV contributed to the end of our relationship. He took it as a free ticket to go out gallivanting around. He was in a lot of denial. I don't know if he was being safe or not. I knew what he was doing. I would confront him, and he kept denying it, saying I was crazy. I really believe that it was him who infected me, but in my heart of hearts it doesn't matter who gave it to who; it's done.

I'm doing pretty good now. I have a son, Robert; he is fourteen. He knows everything. He knew something was up

beatrice

39, diagnosed HIV-positive in 1992, infected through sex

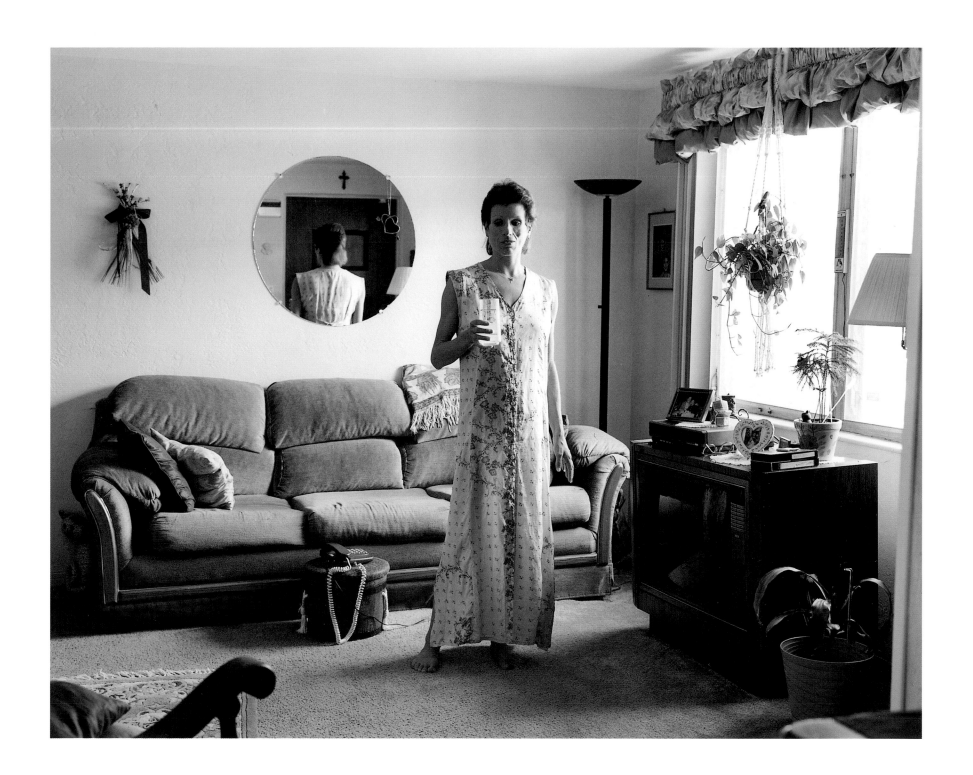

when we found out. I think he was more scared not knowing what was going on than finding out that I was positive. He handles everything okay until I get sick. Then his grades screw up and he monkeys around in school. I have everything set up for him—a trust fund—and he will go live with my mother. He will have everything he needs: my car, the computer, everything he could need except for me.

He won't talk about it. I have tried to talk about me dying. He will not talk to me; not to anybody. We made an agreement that he won't tell anyone because he goes to a Catholic school. I don't want him to be ostracized.

I don't date anyone. I sometimes would like to be with someone. I do well alone. I'm happy with my own company and Robert. If it wasn't for HIV, I would probably pursue another relationship. But when I was sick, I lost like 40 pounds, especially from my face—I'm not very confident with my looks. I go to a women's support group. I don't go to mixed groups. I'm a Catholic. I go to church sometimes; the priest at my church is aware of my situation. My family is very supportive, but they live up north in Rochester, NY.

I used to work at a software company. When I became too ill to work, I told them about my diagnosis. They have offered a lot of moral support. They sent Robert and me on a hot-air balloon ride to Universal Studios and Disneyland. They bought us dinner-theater tickets. They started a trust fund for Robert.

When I was still working full time I started getting temperatures of 104, 105. It would happen in the middle of the day; at night. If Al was home he would throw an ice pack on me and tell me I was heating up the room. I was losing weight, and I couldn't drive because my eyes felt like they were jiggling.

Finally my mother came down to Florida to see what was going on. She saw me and took me in her arms and said you're going to the doctor now. So we went to the doctor. I had MAC and was immediately put in the hospital. They called my family down because they didn't think that I was going to make it. Al and my mom were arguing. She accused him of my deteriorating condition. It was bad.

Somehow I pulled through. My doctor is a real miracle worker. I have managed to keep on some weight, though I still look really thin. I take so many pills a day it's hard to keep count. I get tired all the time. I wake in the morning, do what I have to do—by noon I'm exhausted. I have to take a nap. Later I get up, take care of my son, make dinner, and that's about it. I embroider and go out to the movies sometimes. We have a dollar theater down here and they have some good shows sometimes. I have some really good friends and then I have my best buddy.

She is also infected. I met her through my doctor. He thought that we had a lot in common and we could help each other out. It has worked out really well for both of us. She lives about ten minutes away. We joke around a lot and that really helps to make this thing a little lighter at times. She is gay, and she goes out to bars sometimes. She tells me all about her gay feelings and I talk about my desires for a lasting relationship.

I want to see my son graduate from high school, but I will settle for eighth grade. I want to hang on. Whether it's from a wheelchair or sickbed, I will see my son graduate.

Al and I got divorced in 1994. He still calls. He is almost out of denial. He comes to me when he needs to know something. I truly hated him for what he put me through with the cheating and anger. I don't let that surface for my own benefit.

Before this happened I didn't know anything about HIV. I thought of AIDS as something so foreign. It's a weird thing that happened to other people: gays and drug users. I was neither. I have learned a lot since then, that's for sure.

HIV has not really improved my life, maybe just my cleaning habits. I keep my bathroom and my kitchen cleaner. We always ate good and wholesome, so that is still the same. Spiritually it hasn't forced me onto some spiritual quest.

I'm the same person I was before I was tested. I don't get mad, but I get sad. I don't have a counselor—I try to straighten out when I start crying. I slap myself in the face; tell myself it does no good to cry. I'm past hating this disease. I'm kind of in acceptance. I get sick of taking pills and running to the bathroom with diarrhea, but I'm not feeling too much pain.

alicia mcwilliams

36, HIV-positive since 1988, diagnosed 1991
infected through unprotected sex

I was in Samaritan Village Drug Treatment for about two years. They had a lot of education there about HIV. I can remember I would wake up with night sweats. I would be drenched through my nightgown. I told them I wanted to be tested.

I had a friend there and we would talk about the lifestyle we used to lead and how much more vulnerable we were. It wasn't drug use; it was about being promiscuous. I was petrified. All I heard about HIV was death. You would see people in wheelchairs and looking skeleton-like. I didn't want to get like that. I was very nervous. After listening to all the lectures and all the people with their stories, I just knew in my heart that I was positive.

I made my appointment at the Department of Health in the Bronx. They took the blood and we had to wait 15 days for the test to come back. When he told me, I cried. I cried almost every single day for the next six months.

I get most, if not all, my support from the people at Samaritan Village. All the people there were trying to get clean. We were all from the same background. My girlfriend cried more than I did. There was a staff of HIV coordinators and support groups for people who tested positive. They were really set up to deal with this situation. They treated me like a good family.

When I told my family, my sister made a joke to try and break the tension. She would say, "Hey, you got the Magic Johnson shit." I've tried to educate my family. I know they have learned so much about HIV because of me.

I don't have any children. I was pregnant when I was sixteen and had a partial hysterectomy. Even if I could, I wouldn't want to bring a child into this world with this disease because I might not be around for them. I raised my

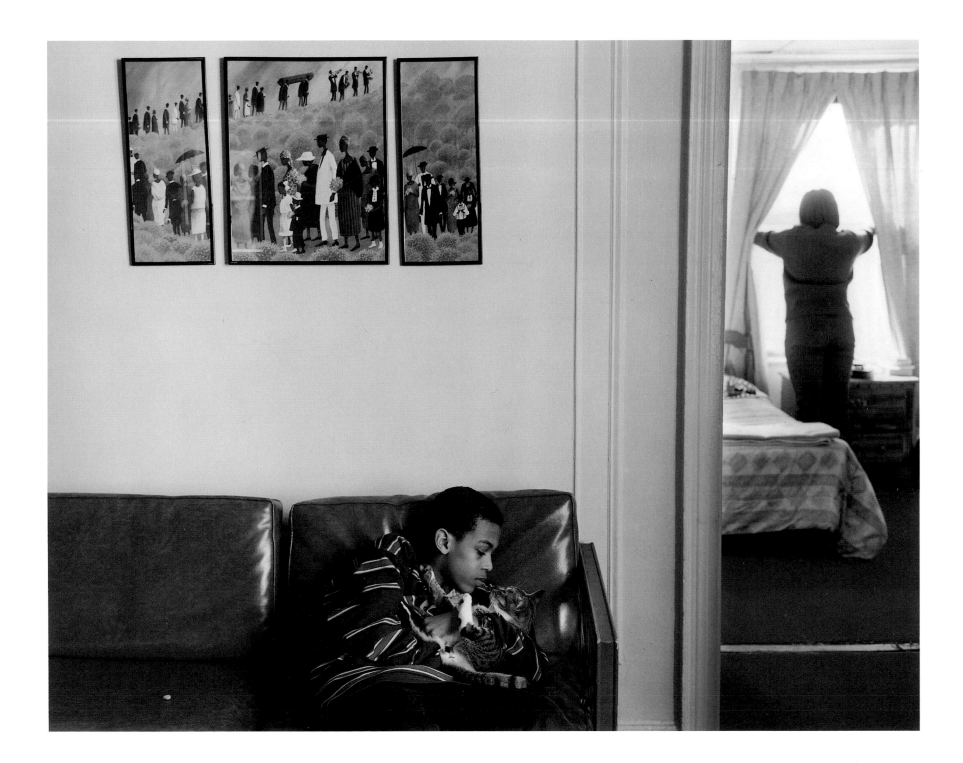

nephew, Hasaan, for two and a half years. It was really beautiful. He just left this October to stay with his father. His mother and I had an agreement that he could stay with me as long as I was well. Even though I wasn't sick, I think that he needed to establish a permanent relationship. He had been shifted around so much. Having Hasaan made me wish that I'd been able to have children, at least just one. It hurt when he left.

I have two cats who I love. Bailey is about seven and her daughter is a year. They are spoiled, but they are my babies.

I was married in 1993. It only lasted three months. I had to get an operation—it wasn't even HIV-related. I had pulled a muscle. My husband just freaked out. He thought I was going to die. He knew going into the marriage that I was HIV-positive; he was negative. I think the operation just brought up a lot of stuff for him.

It made the HIV real. It hit him hard. In the end, our marriage collapsed from his fears.

I date off and on. Some guys you don't want to tell because of rejection. If a man is only looking for one thing (sex), then I really don't want to have anything to do with them. Some guys think that it's a challenge to go out with an HIV-positive woman. Like, "Hey, I survived." And it's another notch on their belt. I really don't know what men think. I have morals, I can be choosy and I choose who I want to deal with. It's important to wait sometimes. My mother never talked to me about sex. I find it fascinating that some of the clients look at me with lust. They say, 'Ooh, you look good.' I say, 'What am I supposed to look like?' I'm a good looking sister—just because I'm positive doesn't mean that I need to look like death warmed over.

For the grace of God, I have only had herpes and thrush. So far, I have been lucky. I have never been sick or in the hospital. My T-cells fluctuate. Right now they are 583. When I broke up with my husband, my mother died at the same time. I lost weight. I got really stressed out and my T-cells went down. I try not to get stressed out anymore.

I enjoy the simple things in life. I can see the beauty in the sky and the trees. Sometimes I think, 'When is my time going to come?' Especially when other people die. Last week I buried a friend. I let people know I'm afraid. Being sick is one of my greatest fears. I know this illness takes people out slow and painfully. I promised myself that I will go out clean and sober. A lot of my friends in recovery that died, went out sober, with dignity. That's how I want it for myself.

I don't feel shame about having HIV. People on my block know because I go out and educate the community. My aunt said one day, 'I know you're living with this, but I didn't know how it impacted on your life.' She asked me to come and speak at her church. People are amazed when I tell them. Especially men. Here they are all ready to just do it, and they don't know what I got. When I tell them, it really leaves them with food for thought.

The government is always experimenting. They might come up with a cure. I think that they could really find an answer if they concentrated all their efforts, at least something better than all the toxic medications they have come up with so far.

I just do vitamins, eat healthy, keep stress low, and have regular checkups. I have a beautiful doctor now. Before, I would have all these doctors. Never the same one. I got tired of it. I just went to a new clinic, and before I signed any papers I told them I wanted a primary caretaker—one familiar face, not six or seven different doctors. It's very important to have the same primary caregiver. That way you don't have to keep explaining and explaining every time you go to the clinic.

I'm an HIV Educator for the Osburn Association. We deal with harm reduction and have a component for substance abuse. I do HIV education for all the groups. We talk about everything. You have to get them to open up their minds. I want people to remember me as someone who worked in the community and helped people. I want to inspire people—let them see that I changed and they can, too, if they want to.

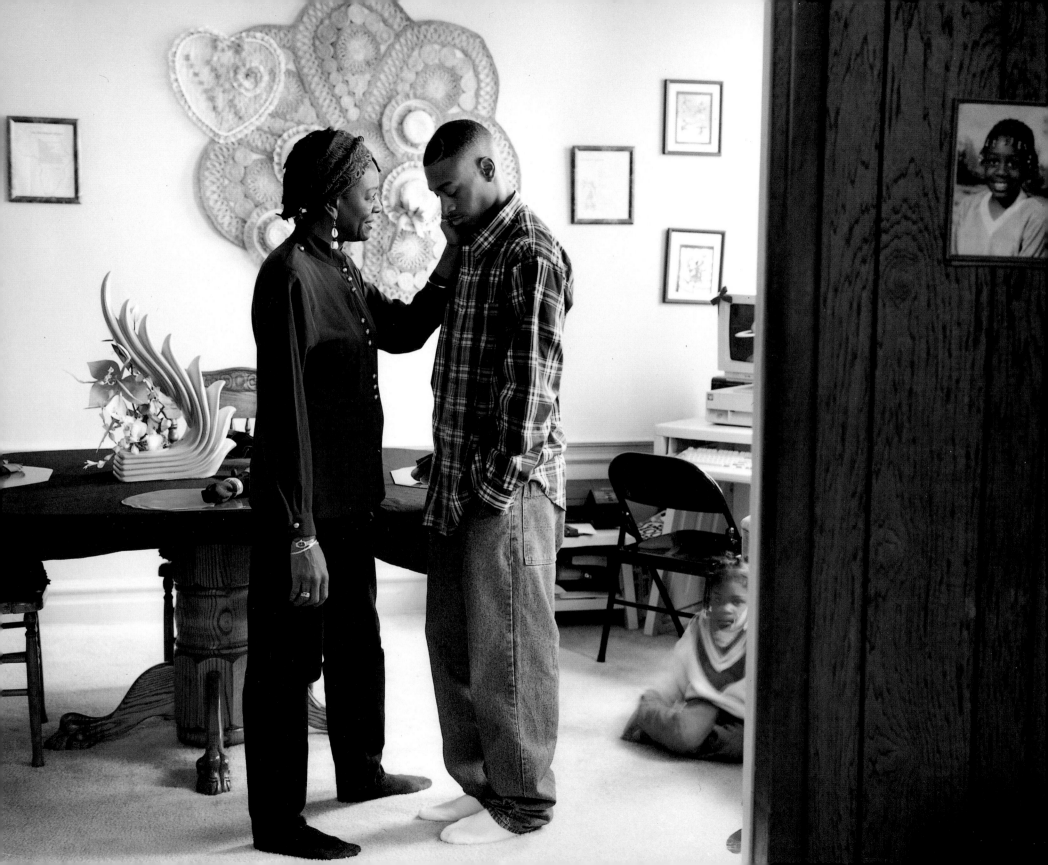

bunny

44, HIV-positive since December 18, 1990,

infected through unprotected sex

I found out I was HIV-positive when I tried to increase my life insurance. One of the requirements was to take a blood test. The insurance company sent some people to my home. They pricked my finger and said that they will get back to me in a couple of weeks. I didn't think much of it. They called me and said that they wanted to take the test again. This time they took two tubes of blood. A couple of days later they called me at work. I was right in the middle of a meeting with 12 attorneys screaming. I took the call, and a man on the other end said that they couldn't give me life insurance because I tested HIV-positive. I was so irritated. I was more mad that he disturbed me at work than the news that I was positive. Actually I wasn't even sure what that meant. I went home to my mother's house and told her that the insurance company refused to increase my policy because I tested HIV-positive. She said, 'Don't worry about it, they make mistakes all the time. Just go get retested.'

I made an appointment with my doctor for the following week. When I went to her office and told her that I wanted to take the HIV test, she said that I didn't fit any of the risk groups—there was no need for me to take that test. Then she asked, 'Who told you to take this test?' I told her the insurance company said I tested positive, and she said that was crazy. She then told me I didn't have anything to worry about—it was a mistake, but we will retest you anyway. I wasn't concerned because she had reassured me that I wasn't at risk. I completely forgot the appointment and didn't show up. She called me at work and said I was supposed to be at her office right now. I said I was busy. She said that I was to be in her office 'at nine A.M. tomorrow, no excuses.' I told my employers that I would be late the next day.

19

I walked into her office and we start arguing back and forth. She wanted me to sit down, and I wanted to stand. Finally, she said I needed to brace myself. I think at that point I knew something was wrong. I sat down. She said I tested positive and my T-cells were 383. She wanted me to start AZT immediately.

She explained that it wasn't a cure but it would help me. She tried to help me understand what HIV was. She said that it was an individual illness. She couldn't tell me when and if I would ever have AIDS. Right now I was HIV-positive and the best thing to do was to take the AZT. She gave me the prescription and I went home.

I still wasn't really clear about what it was I had. I told my mom. She didn't take it too well. She was scared. None of us knew anything about the virus. I think that she went into total denial. The hardest part was to tell my three children. I waited till after the holidays. In February I told Marquita, who is my oldest daughter. She cried and was very upset. Later that evening I told my other daughter. I wasn't able to tell my son till three years later. He was the more emotional of my children. I raised him as a single parent. When I finally did tell him, he already knew something wasn't right. He was worried about who would take care of him if I died. I explained that his sisters would take care of him. They all thought I would be dead in a year.

My T-cells have dropped to 140. I haven't had any serious illness. I feel very fortunate. I take Bactrim, AZT, and 3TC. I have my bad days, but that is normal with everybody.

I stopped working in 1994. I never told people at work. I just resigned from my position. Now I'm collecting disability. I receive $822 a month. My two daughters help me when I need something. It has been six years since I've had the virus, and the biggest problem that has come of it is that I don't make the money that I used to. The financial disability is always a reminder of the virus.

I get up every morning and that is a big deal. I'm getting ready to be a grandma for the fourth time. I am so blessed. I enjoy the moment—especially being with my kids and my grandchildren.

I don't think any of my friends know. Some of my kids' friends know. I gave them that option. I knew how cruel people can be about AIDS. I didn't want them to take it out on my kids. I go to high schools and talk to parents. I also speak to teenagers. One time I was going to speak at my son's school. I asked my son what he thought. He didn't think it was a good idea. Now I don't make a move concerning where I speak unless I clear it with him. He is

I get up every morning and that is a big deal.

I'm getting ready to be a grandma for the fourth time.

I am so blessed.

graduating in June, and I will go speak at his school after he graduates. Very few people in my family know: my mom, the kids, two aunts, and one cousin.

In my life, I never thought of HIV. I had the same attitude that society has. I wasn't doing risky things, so it wasn't going to affect me. I would see programs on TV. I would see it and hear it, but never relate it to myself. I didn't know anyone who had it until after I was diagnosed.

About three years ago, I found out my uncle was dying of AIDS. It was awful. He was my favorite uncle. We weren't supposed to say anything because we weren't supposed to know—it was not discussed. When I told my mom that I wanted to tell the family about my diagnosis, she said, 'No, it's your business.' I needed support, but I wasn't supposed to say anything.

I've tried to help her come to terms with this. I have brought her literature and had some moms whose children have died from AIDS call her. They gave her some numbers she could call for support, but she doesn't call. She thinks it's

a bad dream. I did a lecture once, and a girl from across the street was in the audience. I saw her one day and she said, 'Your mom knows my mom.' She asked how my mom was doing, and I said, 'Not good.' The girl went to see my mom. She told her that she heard me do a lecture. My mom called and asked, 'Why are you doing this? Why are you telling everybody?' She knew I did AIDS education, but didn't know that I told the audience that I was also positive. I tried to explain that it's a form of therapy, and left it at that.

What made me want to go out and speak is I didn't fit any category that people believe are at risk. I wasn't a homosexual, I didn't have lot of lovers, and I never used drugs. I want people to know you can be straight and wind up with this infection.

I've made peace with dying. I don't think I will go before I'm supposed to. I just don't want a whole lot of suffering with illness. I don't want my children to see me suffer. I'm lucky that my kids are grown. I don't have to find someone who will love them as much as I do to guide them correctly.

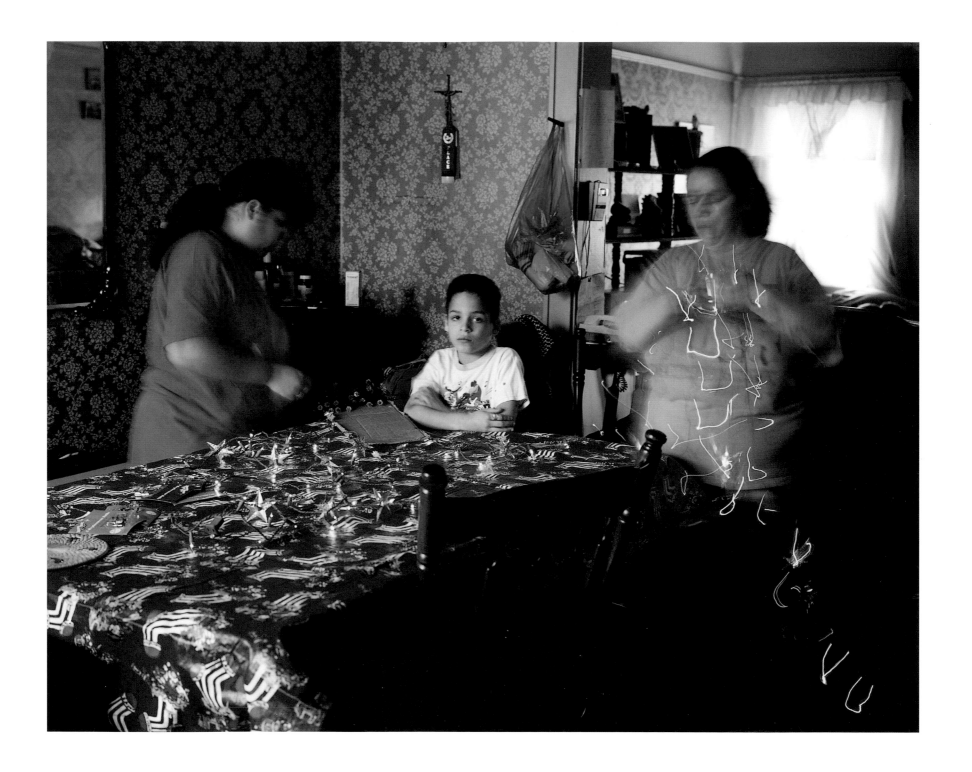

My husband died of AIDS almost three years before I found out I was infected. I was drunk, pregnant, and ready to deliver. I had two bottles of Wild Irish Rose on me to make sure I felt no pain. My baby was born jaundiced, alcoholic, and with the virus. I don't recall them telling me that it could reverse on him. I stayed drunk for about two or three more days then I asked for help because Josh was in the hospital.

I went through detox. It was really hard. They asked me what kind of illnesses I had. I told them: asthma, high blood pressure, and HIV. As soon as I mentioned HIV, the doctors stepped back and said, 'Wait a minute.' They came back covered head to toe in protective gowns, their face and hands covered. I was really scared. I didn't understand HIV at all. I didn't have time to learn.

In a funny way HIV is a blessing. I would be dead or a prostitute by now. I got my life together. I got my kids.

I wasn't able to get my son right away. He was almost nine months old when I was finally together enough to have him with me. He stayed in the hospital. In the rehab and halfway houses I stayed in, we were not allowed to talk about HIV or AIDS. No one was teaching us. I only knew what I heard on the TV or news. It was a no-no because people would get scared. It was only 1987.

I'm married now. I met my husband, William Santiago, in the program. We have been together for nine years; legally for six. William is HIV-negative.

I have been very lucky. I have herpes and thrush and that's it. I want live to see my children graduate and get married. I would like to have some time to enjoy my husband. One thing I want to say to the President, 'Please find a cure. A lot of us are dying fast every day. It's not a joke.'

nilsa ramos "cookie"

40, HIV-positive since 1982, diagnosed in 1987, unsure of how she was infected

barbara causey

47, HIV-positive since September 1987, infected through sex

Keith and I met in 1976. We were both teaching school in Page, Arizona. I taught sixth-grade math, and he taught seventh- and eighth-grade math. He got all my students and he would ask me about them. We were attracted to each other and stayed in touch when I left in 1978.

In 1984 I went to Africa to teach in a missionary school. He sent me a Valentine with a proposal in it. When I got it, I went into shock. We were good friends, but I never thought he would propose. I answered 'yes' in five different languages so he would get the message.

In 1985 I left Africa and I spent four weeks in Albuquerque with Keith. While I was at his house I found a jacket that said "Gay Men's Chorus" on it. I questioned him about it. He explained that he had gotten into that lifestyle through a set of circumstances he didn't have control over. He had been gay for eight years, and then he found the

Lord. The Lord gave him the strength to walk away from it.

We discussed AIDS personally and through our letters. In a letter I asked if he'd be tested before we were married. The night I sent the letter I prayed. I heard the Lord tell me, 'Barbara, I have taken care of you through incest and bigamy, and I will take care of you through this.' I wrote another letter and said, 'You don't have to be tested.' We were married in 1986.

In February of 1987 I became pregnant. When I went to the obstetrician for the preliminary exam, he asked if I ever had a blood transfusion. I had done enough reading to know what they were looking for. I said, 'No, but my husband had been in a high-risk group.' He asked if he would come in to be tested. Kevin went the next week. We waited two months for the results. Finally, the lab called—they were confused. They wanted to know where to send the results because it

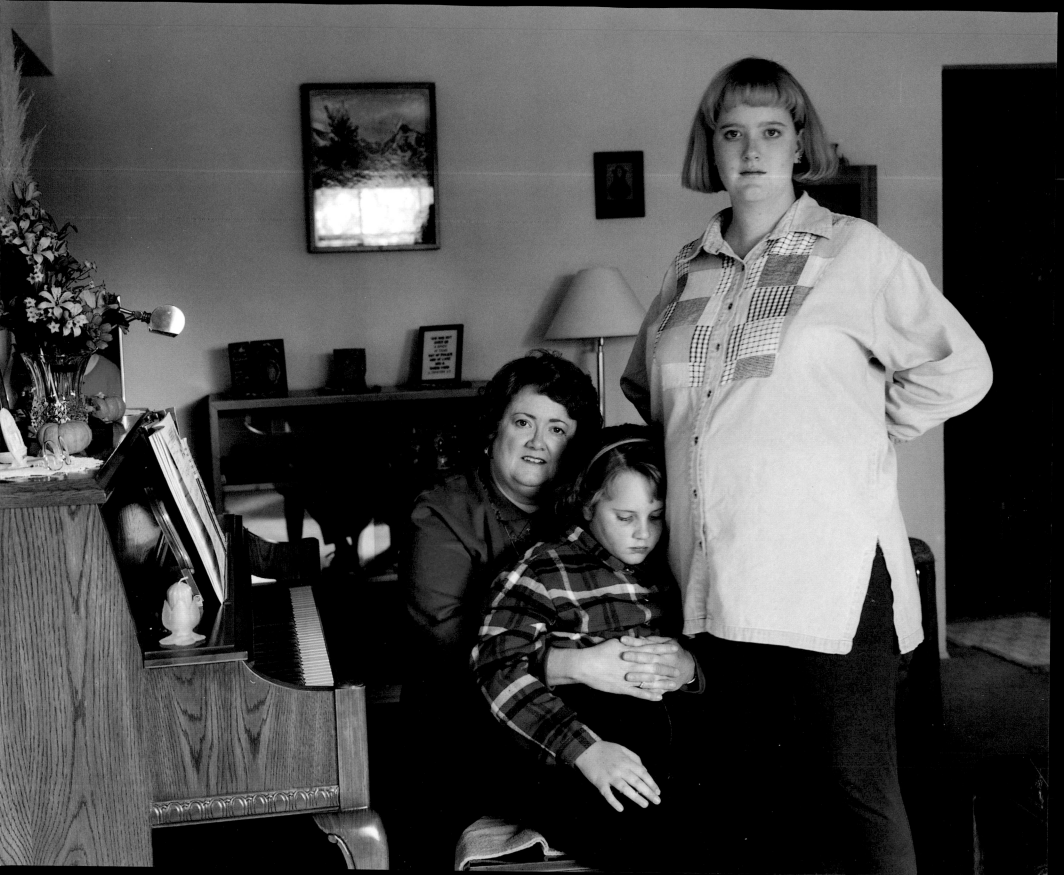

was a gynecologist requesting the test and it was male blood.

When my doctor got the test results, he called me. It was my birthday. I was home alone. He simply called and told me my husband had tested positive. I said, 'Thank you,' and that was the end of the conversation.

I was crushed. I was meeting my husband for lunch. I had to pretend there was nothing wrong. On the way home I stopped at a friend's house and had a good cry. We prayed together. I shared with my husband when he came home.

Keith knew something was wrong. I told him his test was positive. We talked, and he gave me the option to get out of the marriage. I told him our marriage was not just a commitment to him, but to God and him. That was the end of that discussion.

In many ways dealing with Keith distracted me from my own diagnosis. After his test came back positive, they started testing me every three weeks throughout the remainder of my pregnancy. I was negative until the last one before I was due.

When I found out about my diagnosis, I was home alone. The doctor's office called and told me that my test had come back positive. My world fell apart. I was eight-months pregnant. The hospital that I had chosen had never had an HIV birth before, and didn't know if they wanted to start with me. Luckily they accepted me, and my doctor delivered Esther.

My stay was very brief. They made it most uncomfort-

able. They put a yellow contamination sign outside my door. They would not let me take a shower on my floor. None of my food trays were taken out of my room till the room was decontaminated. The staff would come in fully dressed in mask, gown, and goggles to bring me food. They put the baby in isolation, but there were not enough nurses to watch over her so they put her in my room. The pediatric nurse acted as if she never touched a baby before because she was so afraid.

They tested her in the hospital.

They didn't ask me or tell me. They just called me when she was four days old and said, 'Your daughter tested positive.' That was all they said—and hung up.

I tried calling my husband and my pastor, but no one was home. Finally, I got a hold of a social worker. She told me there were so few HIV births that the statistics were skimpy. All she knew was 50 percent die before a year old, 25 percent are sickly and die as teens, and another 25 percent somehow end up testing negative after a year or two.

I cried. I never thought I would see my baby grow past a year. I think that was the low point in our lives. I prayed every time I changed her diapers that God would spare her.

When Esther was a year old, the pediatric specialist called me on the phone. She said, 'I know I shouldn't tell you this on the phone, but I couldn't wait. Esther's test came back negative.'

Again I tried my husband and the pastor, but no one was available. So I called the social worker. She was so elated that she was saying it out loud to anyone that was listening. 'Esther is negative!' It was like Esther had been born all over again.

During the time that Keith was sick, my doctor told me I didn't have to worry. He said there won't be any problems for about five years. Within two years, my T-cells were below half of what they should have been. I knew I needed to take AZT. Keith encouraged me and helped me to get started. I didn't have the same reactions that he did—just a great deal of nausea. I was on it nine months. I couldn't eat, cook, or go to the grocery store, so I stopped. I was off for six months and my count went down. I went back on it at the time when Keith was so sick; my count stayed the same.

At the clinic they found out Keith's T-cell count was below 200. They started him on AZT. He was one of the people who had a bad reaction. He was on it for a year. He became extremely anemic. He was getting transfusions every ten days. Finally they took him off AZT. There was nothing else to try. He briefly regained his health. But then he started to get one opportunistic infection after another. He was put on medicines for each one. By the time he died,

he was taking 21 medications. He had developed a pill ulcer in the esophagus. He could no longer eat because of the pain. He basically starved to death.

Keith died in May 1991. We were married just shy of five years. He was very sick the last year and a half. I was his primary caregiver. Debbie, my daughter, ended up doing most of Esther's care giving. It was a very difficult time. I had to learn how to put in an IV. I watched the man I love deteriorate. He went from being a healthy 155-pound man to less than 90 pounds.

There was a peace with Keith in the end. The day before he died, he couldn't move or talk. He rolled over and smiled at me. I asked, 'Honey are you all right?' He said, 'I hear Jesus calling and I'm happy.' He passed away 12 hours later.

My friends were worried because I didn't cry, but Keith and I had said our good-byes. I knew where Keith was going. There was a lot of grieving while he was sick. I cried a lot in the shower where no one could hear me. I didn't want Keith to know how upset I was.

I'm now on AZT, 3TC, and Crixivan. My viral load was 15,000; last month it was below 200. My T-cells have not responded. They are currently at 138. I have not been ill. God has kept me well and there are many people praying for me. They give me the strength to keep going.

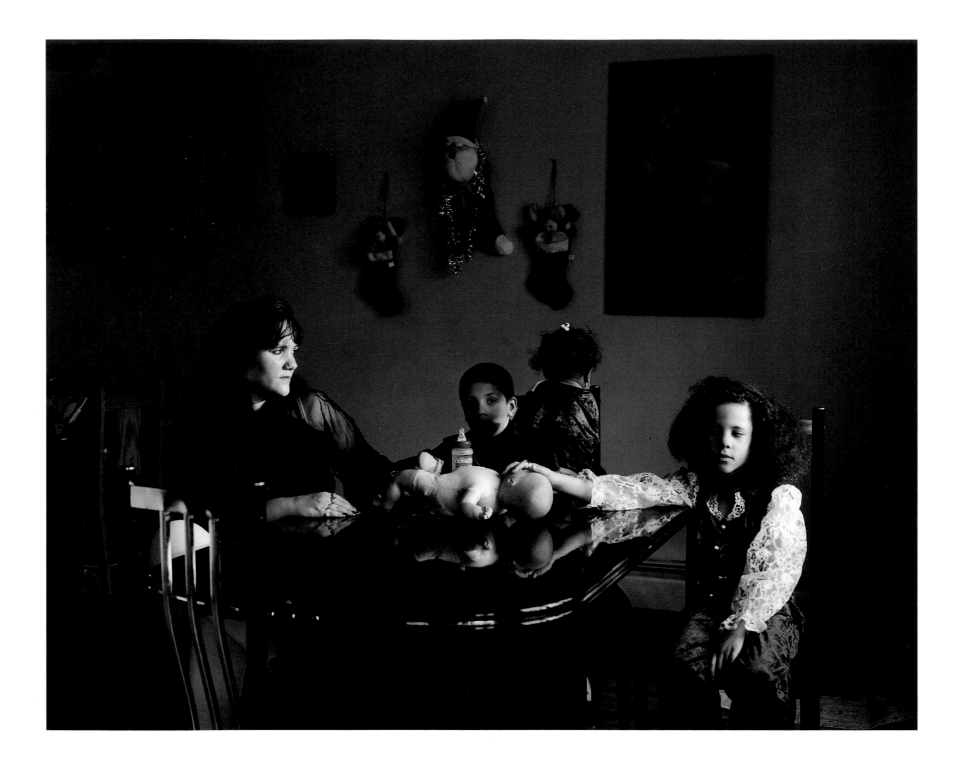

I don't see this disease as a death sentence, but sometimes when I get sick I get real scared . . . I'm at the point where it's like, 'Oh boy, here I go again.' Very nonchalant. I have been through a lot of illnesses—some real close calls. Last year the doctors thought I was going to lose my eyesight. I was walking around in a daze. Even though I knew it was not life-threatening, I couldn't bear the idea of not being able to see—I might as well be dead. I need my eyesight. Take my hearing, take my arm, just let me see. Another time I had PCP pneumonia. I wanted to die. I lost control over my bowels, I had a fever of 105; I told the nurse, 'Just give me something, or kill me.' It was horrible. Right now I have cervical dysplasia. They have been doing biopsies and I'm at the point where I want them to just give me a hysterectomy, but they say I'm too weak. As far as medication goes, I'm not an antiviral kind of person, I never wanted to take AZT. But right now I'm on a combination therapy plus protease inhibitor, and I'm hoping for the best. I have about 15 T-cells left.

The funny thing is that I gained weight. I must have gained fifty pounds, I'm heavier than I have ever been. People never believe that I'm sick. Everyone says, 'You look so good, so healthy.' They think if you're not all wasted, you're not sick. I really hate when people say that I look so good, like, 'It's okay, she looks good,' and they can dismiss you as not really being sick. They feel better. In reality, I will probably look good till I'm dead. I can see everyone at my funeral saying, 'But she looked so good.'

It seems to me that women just don't waste the same way as men. All the women in my group are heavy. I don't like being heavy. I'm still a woman and would like to fit into size 5 jeans again. And let me tell you, lugging this weight up

april drew

29, diagnosed HIV-positive in 1989, infected through sex

the stairs is no easy feat, especially when you're feeling sick. My doctor doesn't think I should diet. He comes into the office with a soda and a candy bar and asks, 'Do you want some?' It's weird. He is overweight, too, and maybe my fat makes him more comfortable. Sometimes I think I really would like to lose weight, but I usually end up saying something like, "Oh, I'm sick, let me eat what I want."

I have a boyfriend; he is HIV-positive. I met him through an HIV-positive support network. We usually practice safe sex but not all the time. I never tell my doctor if we don't practice safe sex because I know that I will get a long lecture about passing the virus back and forth. We do the best we can, but we are only human. This is actually the first person I have had sex with, besides the man that I was infected by, who is HIV-positive. All the other men I have been with are HIV-negative. I have never had a problem with having dates or relationships. When I would tell them that I was HIV-positive, they would just take it in stride. I guess that tells you where men's heads are at when it comes to sex. I had men tell me that they didn't want to use any protection with me, even though they knew I was positive.

I don't trust a man who won't use protection. I know what I have, but I don't know what he may have, and whatever it is, I don't want it. I have always practiced safe sex with people that are negative, but there were a few accidents—that is how I had my last daughter.

I decided to keep the baby. I had to put up with a lot of negative input for wanting this baby, especially by the gynecologist that was treating me. For the first 24 weeks, every single visit she would say, 'It's not too late to have an abortion.' But I told her I had made up my mind—this is what I want. I felt pushed by her. My mother was also against me having the baby; she was really upset. She felt that the baby was going to be sick. She didn't want to get attached to the baby because it was probably going to die. She would say, 'Why bring a sick child into the world?' Even though we didn't know she wasn't going to be infected, it seemed like everyone assumed that would be the case.

After she was born we had to wait five months before we would know if she was going to be positive or convert to being negative. It was hard when I found out that she was definitely HIV-positive. I became distant with her. I didn't think I could take the pain of losing her. But that lasted for

I don't trust a man who won't use protection.

I know what I have, but I don't know what he may have,

and whatever it is, I don't want it.

only a week or so. I mean, she's my little girl.

It was really difficult in the beginning. She kept getting smaller and smaller. I was afraid she was going to die. She had thrush, diarrhea, and pneumonia; all this before she was five months old. Now she is two, and doing really well. She is a chubby, happy little girl. I have no regrets at all that I had her.

It's my children, friends, and cats that really keep me going. I think once you're sick for so long, you almost get used to it. You get used to the pain and weakness to the point that it almost feels normal—you forget what it's like to be healthy. All my closest friends know I'm HIV-positive, but I don't think I would go on national TV and tell the world. I never did drugs. I didn't even smoke cigarettes. I got this through sex. I tell people, because so many people still do not believe that they can get this thing, especially women. I had to learn the hard way, so anytime I get a

chance I try to squeeze in a little lesson about safe sex.

The first few years I didn't tell anybody, but when I stopped fearing it myself I started to be able to tell other people. In the beginning, I feared being rejected, shunned, and having people ostracize my children.

I remember when I was first diagnosed. My friend made me this big dinner, and I watched to see where she put my plates and utensils. Did she wash them different? Did she put them separate from the rest of her other things? I was surprised that she didn't. I watched my family to see if they disinfected the toilet bowel after I used it. But it seemed that I was the one who was most afraid: not of infecting anyone, but just of how friends and family would feel about me.

My two oldest children know. Justin and Shauni are ten and eleven. They have known for two years. They know how I contracted the disease; they know how you get it. They could probably teach people a few things.

susan

28, HIV-positive since 1988, diagnosed in September 1994
infected through sex

I went to Boston's Children's Hospital to see if Anna's bones were in place. When they took the X-rays, they look at everything. By fluke really they saw that she had an enlarged heart. I took her to see a cardiologist. He recommended putting her in the hospital. While we were in the hospital, the doctor felt that my daughter's symptoms were very characteristic of HIV infection. He said we should get tested.

My first reaction was anger at him for suggesting this. He asked me, 'You don't have HIV do you?' That made me even more angry. If I had that kind of information I would mention it. All the interns were asking if I had ever slept with anyone who had AIDS. I wanted to grab my daughter and run out of there.

I was very worried about my daughter. We both took the test to rule out HIV. We were supposed to get the blood tests back in two days. We didn't hear from them for a month.

In the meantime my husband went to a place that gave you your results in one hour. His test came back negative, and that kind of gave me hope that the doctors were wrong. When we didn't hear right back from the first doctor, I decided to take my daughter to an infectious disease specialist. Initially, he gave us optimism. When he looked at my daughter's records, he said, 'It could be HIV but it could be other things also.' He gave us another HIV test. He told us we would have our answer in two days. I had said to him, 'Look, I'm not suicidal. You can give me the results over the phone.' I called two days later, and he said he didn't have the results just yet. He asked if I could come into his office the next day. Right then I kind of knew that the tests had come back positive.

We went to his office the next day. When he told us, I really had no emotions. The doctor said, addressing my

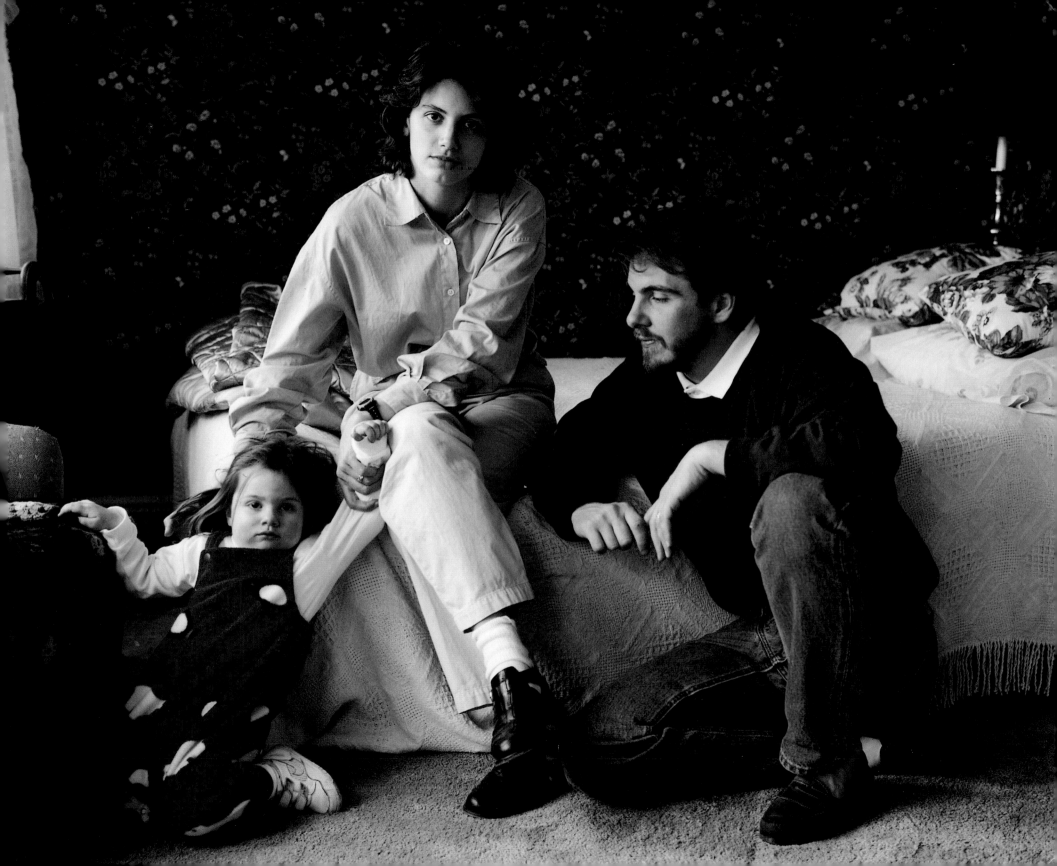

husband, 'I have good news for you.' But we already knew his test was negative. Turning to me, he said, 'I don't have such good news for you. The test came out positive for both you and your daughter.' When he started with the good news–bad news stuff I really thought maybe it wasn't HIV. I was holding my husband's hand. His voice started to tremble badly. The color drained from his face.

That was about a year and a half ago. When I first found out, I was very emotional. I dropped out of school. I acted like a machine. I did what I had to do for my daughter, Anna. Once that was settled, I took care of myself.

My daughter is a lot healthier than she was. She doesn't get as many ear infections, and she has gained weight. The thrush comes back once in a while. She doesn't know what she has. She has another health problem that they didn't diagnose until after the HIV. She has cerebral palsy. At first they just thought that she didn't want to let go of my hand. But then it became apparent that she had real trouble walking.

Anna is outgoing and friendly. She is the most intuitive child. I know a lot of children are sensitive, but I really think that she has this sixth sense when it comes to other people's feelings. She knows exactly how you're feeling. If she senses that something is wrong, she will come over and pat you on the back and give you a hug.

She has had so many tests done to her that she knows something is wrong. She has had a spinal tap, an MRI, and a catheter up her urethra so many times. With her cerebral palsy, she goes to school for therapy. They don't know how HIV affects her cerebral palsy, really. She has a mild case.

When I see how she struggles to walk it reminds me she has AIDS. It screams out at me, "AIDS!" It doesn't say, "cerebral palsy," it says, "AIDS." Sometimes, a lot of times, I feel really angry and cheated; mostly just cheated.

I always thought I should have been tested before. I dated a man once who, in retrospect, acted very strange. He wasn't working when I met him even though he had his own company. I always thought that was odd. One time I got hepatitis—he called me in the hospital and he told me he loved me. This was really inappropriate for our relationship. Earlier in the relationship, he would always say, 'Don't I look good?' like he needed reassurance. He definitely knew he had HIV when we were together. He even mentioned it once. He said it was God's way of punishing people for being too promiscuous. This was 1988. Another time, he said, 'Oh, I have AIDS.' Then he said he was just kidding. I said, 'I don't kid about things like that.' When I tried to get in touch with him about a year and a half later, his telephone was disconnected. I'm assuming he is dead.

I'm angry at him. I would like to find out why he did what he did. He was definitely sleeping around a lot. He had one steady girlfriend and tons of other girls that he was seeing. I would like to get in touch with his girlfriend. I was dating him thinking he was breaking up with this woman. I know she didn't know anything. She used to come in through the pharmacy where I worked to pick up her birth-control pills. Obviously they weren't using condoms, either.

I have 150 T-cells. I used to be afraid of dying. Now it feels surreal, like this is really not a problem for me. Besides taking all the pills, I feel like I don't really have anything wrong with me. I'm okay. I'm really healthy, though things happen to me. I get yeast infections all the time and fungus on my toenails. I get really tired.

My husband, Roy, is very supportive. We have been married for four years. He has never said to me anything like he can't take this anymore. But I know this is difficult for him. It really hurts him to not see his daughter walk. It's the 'not knowing if we will be around' that scares him the most.

We still have sex. In the beginning we had a

problem with it. Really, I had a problem with it. If my gums were bleeding, we couldn't kiss. And I would always be getting yeast infections because I was so sensitive. I would think of all the consequences and that would turn me off; it

still does. Roy would claim he wasn't afraid of getting infected. He pushed for us to have sex. I would go for months not wanting to do it. I know that it was very frustrating for him. Now we have protected sex, but it limits us. I fantasize about having unprotected sex.

It was really difficult telling my mother. My mom was really depressed for a long time. I finally had to say, 'Mom you have to deal with this. You have to get it together.' I have a brother and we're really close. He doesn't talk about it. My family can't deal with it. They are ashamed.

Roy's family is much more open. They tell everyone they know. They send information, offer support. They are really great about it. They are not ashamed about it. My husband's uncle died of AIDS, so they are familiar with HIV.

When I'm really down, I feel like, 'Oh my God, Anna isn't going to have a long life. Neither one of us is going to have a long life.' Then I see my doctor, and I think that everything is going to be all right—no problem. With all these new drugs there's a lot of hope. It might seem hard, but in the long run it will be okay.

It's almost like AIDS gives me some kind of freedom. Like it can't get any worse, so go for it. I have nothing to lose. Risks are not so risky, especially emotional risks. Before HIV, I wasn't very assertive. I say what I feel now. AIDS has definitely made me a lot stronger.

patricia annichiarico

31, HIV-positive since 1986, diagnosed in 1990, infected through IV drugs or sex

My husband, Kevin, died four years ago. We were together five years. He was Irish and Scottish—really handsome. We were friends for about a year before we got married. We played on the same softball team in Central Park.

The first year and a half that we were together was great. Neither of us were doing drugs. Then Kevin got really sick. He started getting high by himself. He would sneak around behind my back. He did not want me to know what was going on. Once I insisted that I go with him. We went to this place and he copped heroin. That time he only sniffed it. I wanted to do it with him. I had started to feel left out of his life. I thought that getting high together would be the answer. The next time I went with him, I saw that he was using a needle. I really freaked out. I said, 'Pick that or me.' He chose. I went and got a cab home. Eventually, I just went along and started getting high with him.

After that, we both got so involved in drugs that the relationship really suffered. He never told me he was infected. I think he was in a lot of denial. By not telling me, he didn't have to face it himself. Whenever he became ill, with pneumonia or something, he would just go to the emergency room. He always went to a different ER, so that they wouldn't know that he was positive. He didn't see a doctor for his condition at all until the end. He would try to hide it from me. Like one time he was in Lenox Hill Hospital with pneumonia. They had a sign on the door about infectious body fluids. He said that the place was crowded, and they had to put him in this room with a guy who had AIDS.

He eventually got PML, which is a degenerative disease of the brain. He didn't do anything about it. He eventually became disoriented; what I guess you would call dementia. Before the drugs, he was a really intelligent man. He used to

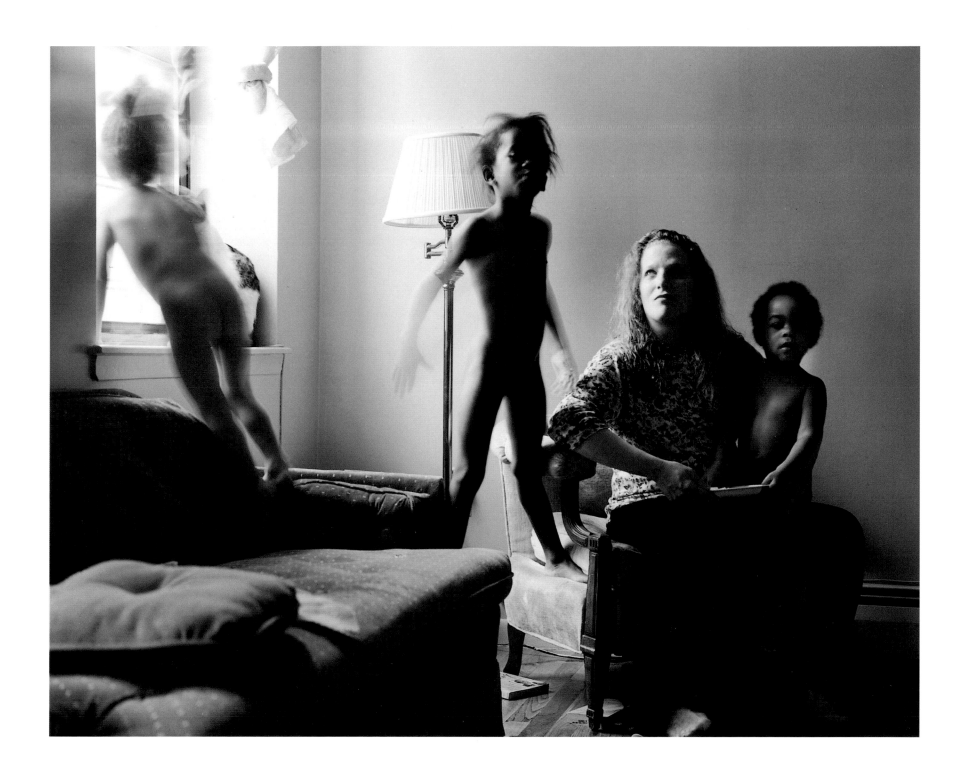

have lots of interests. He liked hunting in the Adirondacks. He was really into rifles and had a pretty good collection. All legal, of course. After the PML started to affect his thinking, he would wander around the neighborhood with his guns. One time he got arrested. When I went to get him out, the police told me I was lucky that they didn't shoot him. I said, 'You mean you would have shot him in the foot?' They said, 'No, that is only on TV. We're trained to shoot to kill when someone is walking around threatening people with a gun.'

He did all kinds of crazy things. In the end we had to have someone watch him all the time.

He spent his last five months tied to a bed in a hospice on Roosevelt Island. He had to stay tied up because he would try to get out of the bed. This was a problem because he could no longer maintain his balance and would fall right down. I would come and visit him and he would be all twisted up because he had been trying to get out. He didn't know where he was, but he always recognized me. He would say, 'I'm so glad you're here, untie me!'

This hospice was a Medicaid hospice. Most of the patients were on drugs or were homeless. The treatment there was awful—awful. They didn't take care of the patients at all. They only changed the diapers twice a day. If someone had a bowel movement in between, they just had

to sit in their mess till it was 'diaper changing' time. I changed so many diapers while I was there. Most of the patients had no one. It just seemed like these people were unwanted by anyone, including the staff.

After Kevin died, I went home to stay with my family in New Jersey. That's where I ended up taking the test. I had hoped that I was negative, but I kind of knew that I was positive. Kevin's doctor had always urged me to get tested. She had been really nice to me, so when I found out that I was positive, I called her. She checked my T-cells. They were only 180, but I had no symptoms.

Something happened to me when I found out I was positive. I was able to find something in me that wanted to live. I didn't want to get high to the end. I didn't want to die being lonely and depressed. I started to clean up my act. I went on methadone and volunteered at the Gay Men's Health Clinic (GMHC).

I was working at the Child Life division of GMHC. There was a client there who was pregnant. She had just been arrested for possession of crack and had to go to jail for a month. She needed someone to take care of her baby until she got released. I met her and she liked me, so I took her baby. The baby was only a day old and had been born HIV-positive. When the mother got out of jail, she was still using crack. I got temporary custody for a year. A social worker got me into a foster agency so I could begin the process of becoming a foster mother to Dawn, the little girl. They felt that it was okay that I was HIV-positive because the baby was still positive. But all that changed when Dawn seroconverted to HIV-negative. Now it has become really hard to convince them that I would be a good choice. They say that everything is against me: I'm HIV-positive, single, and on a methadone program. This month we went to court and the mother forfeited her rights as guardian to Dawn. It's a really slow process. I'm a little scared, to put it lightly. Especially when they told me it was a long shot. But I had to snap out of it. I have had her for two years. I just have to believe that in the end she will be mine legally.

Dawn is the greatest thing that ever happened to me. She is my little miracle. I really believe she is meant to be with me.

I hate being on methadone. It's also a major obstacle with the adoption. Every time that I tell my doctors I want to detox, they're dead set against it. The doctors say that methadone actually helps your immune system. They were telling me that most long-term survivors, who I guess were IV drug users, were on methadone. I said, 'If the stuff is that good, why aren't they giving it out as medication?' Not a day goes by that I don't wish that I could get off it.

Most of my emotional support comes from my counselor at the clinic and Sylvia, my social worker. My brothers have been real good to me also. HIV has been really hard on the rest of my family. They're 'suburban' people. They're very concerned about how things look. God, when I brought Dawn home last Christmas they almost died because she's black. I can see how I could have been just like them if I hadn't recovered spiritually and emotionally. They're horrified at my past as an addict and my HIV diagnosis.

There are two dreams that I have. One is getting off methadone and the second is parting with the DES. They treat you so badly down there, like you're a piece of garbage. I would just love to be able to support myself and my child.

I hope to keep Dawn, see her go to college, and raise her with good self-esteem. I know that this might be really hard. It's obvious to everyone that she isn't my biological child. People ask me all the time, like on the bus, 'Is she your kid?' And now she is starting to understand. I can see that this hurts her. Kids in school can be really mean. I just hope that I can teach her to be strong and proud of who she is.

I haven't fully realized all my potential. I used to think I was useless, and I have found out that I have some gifts. I'm very good with children. Everybody says so. I want to do something with children. I want to go to school so I can teach. I think it would be incredible to have a job that you love.

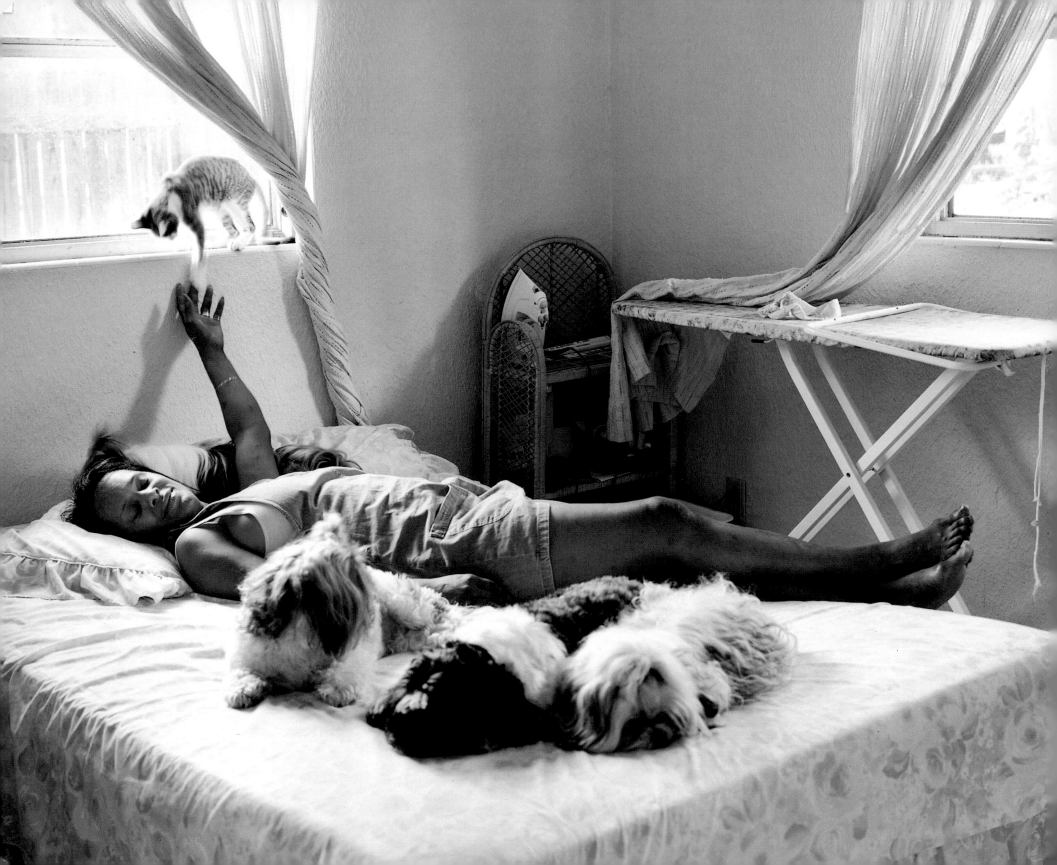

I had a blood transfusion twice. I was an intravenous drug user and I was very promiscuous, so I don't know how I was infected. It doesn't really matter.

I found out because I had stuck my hand with a pin. Overnight it turned green. I stayed in the hospital for 28 days. My hand was virtually green. They packed it twice and it still wasn't getting better. They asked me about my lifestyle and said maybe I should take an HIV test. I said, 'Sure.' I had very little information about HIV so I didn't have any fear.

A few days later, a priest, two nuns, and a doctor came in my room. They told me my test came back HIV positive. They prayed for me. Then they told me to eat a lot of lettuce. I will never forget that. They scared me to death praying over me. I can laugh now about the lettuce. I was depressed for a couple of minutes, then a nurse came in and touched me. When she touched me I knew it couldn't be all bad. I couldn't give it to anyone by touching.

At the time I was dating Kevin, who is now my husband. He was the first person I told. He told me not to worry. I would be okay. It never bothered him. He took an HIV test and it was negative. After that he took one every six months. Around 1990 he stopped being regular about taking the test until he stopped altogether.

In 1994 we went to get insurance for the house. They came right to the house to take his blood. I didn't even know it was an HIV test. The insurance company never told him his test came back positive. They just sent him a letter saying they could not give us insurance. It was awful the way they did it. They registered his positive result with the state of Florida, and the Health Department put a note on our door saying it was urgent that we contact them. By

meredith

41, diagnosed HIV-positive in 1985,
source of transmission—unknown

I don't think there will be a cure in my lifetime.

I do think there will be a regimen

that will help you live a reasonably normal life.

I know this because I'm taking it now.

then we knew. I went with Kevin. They didn't want me there. Kevin insisted. He said, 'Look this is my wife. If you're going to tell us that I tested HIV positive, we know.'

We never practiced safe sex. We tried it a few times. Kevin didn't like the condoms. I'd watched my husband put a condom on a full erection, and then he would lose it. He would tell me that he didn't fear HIV. He would say, 'I look at you and see you can survive.'

After he tested positive I had to work on my guilt. I went to therapy and group sessions. I had to come up with a way to deal with it. I love my husband. He made his choice. The results were inevitable. It's just the way life is. People in relationships with people who are HIV positive have this bizarre loyalty like, "I love her and I don't care." If a man is with someone who is infected, they're in it for the duration. They know the deal. It doesn't make it right, it doesn't make it wrong, it's a choice.

HIV is not the end of life. I work a full-time job. We

can't have children so we compensate with the dogs. We don't let it affect us. We eat well, pay the mortgage. Everything after that is a gift.

Kevin has his own way of dealing with his disease. We have different doctors. His treatment is none of my business. We are comfortable with our diseases. Every so often we talk about it, but not all the time.

We are both taking protease inhibitors. From the beginning I've never had over 300 T-cells. I've never been sick. The only things I've had are herpes and yeast infections.

Kevin has never been sick. He is 219 pounds and over six feet tall. His T-cells are 600. I asked him to loan me a couple. He said, 'No.'

I have a really good network. Kevin

doesn't have any support apart from me. I don't think it's good for him. I don't mind, but I know it helps me to have a larger circle of support. I tell my girlfriends all the time about HIV. The results of what you call "fun." I tell them you don't want to be in the place I'm in. I deal with this because I have to, but I would rather not be here. I don't think I'm being punished. I'm one of the thousands who ended up being infected. It could have been cancer; it could be diabetes; it happens to be HIV.

My mom and sister are the only ones that know. I want to tell my older brother, Maxwell, but I want to tell him face to face. He needs to see me when I tell him so he knows I'm all right.

My younger brother is also positive. He is very angry about it. He would say, 'Why buy a house because you won't be here to enjoy it.' He blames me for his disease. He idolized me when he was a kid. He did drugs but I believe he got it from sex. He is gay, though he will deny it. He was raped in Easton Military Academy and he thinks that's what started him having sex with men. We're not really on good terms. I love him but he's very negative and that's not good for me.

I don't think there will be a cure in my lifetime. I do think there will be a regimen that will help you live a reasonably normal life. I know this because I'm taking it now. I think the knowledge more than the medicine keeps me feeling good. I started taking AZT in 1991. It has done

well for me. My T-cells went from 3 to 416. I will not go off AZT. I've been taking it for five-and-a-half years. I've only stopped once, and my T-cells dropped. I know my body. I'm consistent. I think that's important. In 1990 I stopped drinking, smoking reefer, and cigarettes. I get my exercise from my job. It's very physical—I work at a giant retail store.

My husband's family doesn't know.

They are from Wisconsin. I went to AIDS Manasota, a conference for people with AIDS. When I came home, they asked where I had been. I told them I went to an AIDS conference. They asked, 'Why did you go?' I tell them I take women I sponsor from Alcoholics Anonymous. I try to help them be open. His dad said, 'Those people are really dirty. You can never drink behind them. They will open a can of beer, drink from it and then close it back up and pass it on to you.'

That's when my husband will say, 'Sweetie you need to go and get dressed.' Sometimes I can't believe how ignorant people can be. This man has no concept. Every time he comes to visit he gives me a big kiss on the lips. I give him a hug and I smile to myself. I do worry about when this book comes out and how it will affect him.

karri stokely

30, diagnosed HIV-positive in June 1996, unsure of transmission

I'm not sure of how I was infected. I've had unprotected sex. I worked as an EMT and was splashed and spattered with everything and experienced needle sticks on a number of occasions. I had a blood transfusion in 1984. I'm not in contact with any of the men from my past and I have never been notified about a possible contamination from the blood I received. So I plain don't know.

I understand people are interested in how I was infected. It helps them form opinions on you. We need to put labels on people according to how they look or who we think they are and how they conduct their lives. People decide if you're worthy of their empathy depending on how you were infected. It's really judgmental. Like you deserve it if you slept with 50 men, but you're an innocent if it was only one. People have turned it into a moral issue. When it comes right down to it, it really doesn't matter. In reality it's a deadly disease that doesn't discriminate.

I delivered my second child, Jack, by C-section. I got a staph infection that became septic and then acute toxic hepatitis.

The doctors said the infections were caused by an allergic reaction from the antibiotics. While I was still in the hospital recovering from these infections they found CMV in my blood. I didn't know what it was. They told me that 80 percent of the population carried this disease and didn't know it. I shouldn't worry about it. Later I found out that it's an opportunistic illness that defines AIDS.

It took about two and half months for me to heal from the C-section. I still didn't feel any better. I thought it was taking me too long to bounce back. I couldn't get through the day.

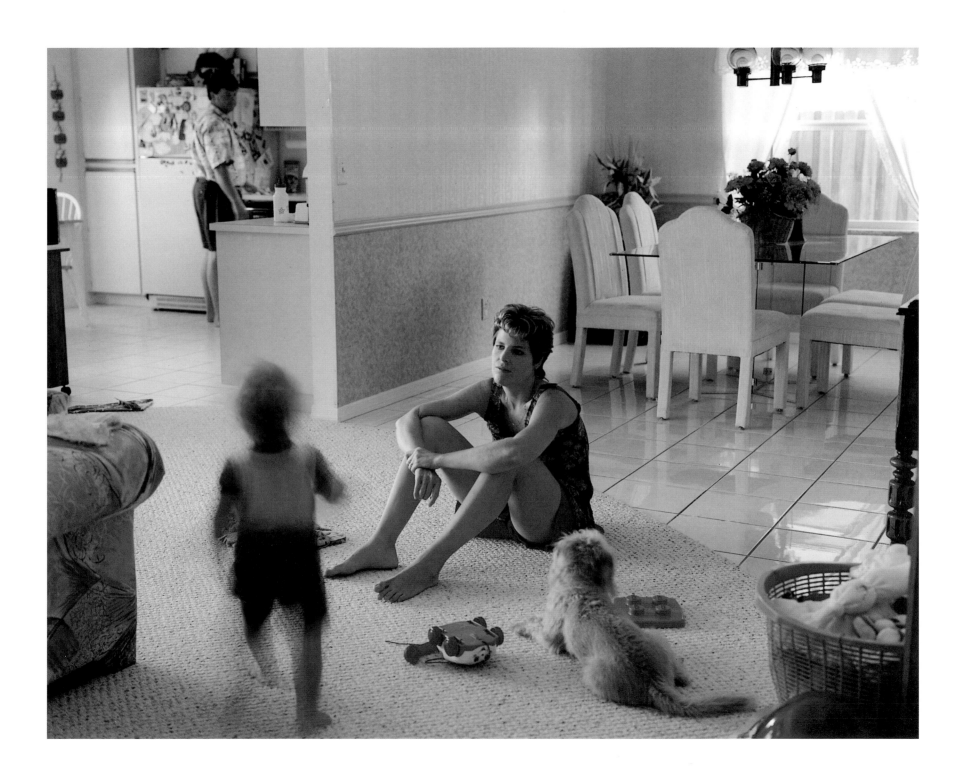

I went to an internal medicine doctor and told him what was happening. I was constantly having headaches and body aches. He said it was probably the CMV and I was too busy. He felt I needed a vacation. I was not happy with his suggestions. His nurse took me aside and suggested that I see an infectious disease specialist because of the CMV. So I went to the infectious disease specialist and told him the whole story. I brought all my lab work, medical records, and hospital birth records.

He asked if I ever had an HIV test.

I said I didn't think so. I remember him asking me some personal questions about my sex life. I told him that I had been married for seven years and he dropped his inquiry pretty quick. I could tell he didn't want to probe.

He gave me some Prozac and told me to come back in six weeks. He was making it seem like I wasn't feeling good because I was depressed. If nothing was abnormal on the tests then everything would go away once my depression was alleviated with the Prozac. I tried to tell him I was depressed because I was sick, not sick because I was depressed. I'm not a depressed person. I wasn't happy with his Prozac suggestion. From there I went to see a hematologist.

By now it was almost a year that I had been feeling ill. This doctor was really thorough. He read all the charts and asked a thousand questions. He thought it was my liver. At the end of the visit he said to me, 'Have you ever had an HIV test?' I said, 'I don't think so.' He said, 'Surely they did one when you were pregnant?' I didn't remember that ever coming up. He suggested that we do one just to rule it out; to cover all the bases. I asked, 'Do you think that's what it is?' He said, 'No I don't, but we should just take the test and make sure.' I really didn't give it much thought.

I was supposed to come back in three weeks. The office called three days later and asked if I could come that day, literally within hours. The nurse tried to sound happy but I could tell that something was definitely wrong. I had worked in medicine long enough to know they were not calling me in to say hello.

I called my husband at work. I told him to come home right away. I was in tears. I didn't suspect it was HIV, but I did think it was something terrible. When we arrived at the doctor's office we were immediately ushered into his office. The doctor came into the room looking at the floor, shaking his head and said, 'Your HIV test came back positive.' We were stunned. We both started crying. The doctor just watched and never said a word. Finally he stood up and said you have to go back and see your infectious disease specialist and basically ushered us to the door. I felt like he wanted us out of there.

My health has improved. I feel

a lot better. Before I had bad days and really, really bad days;

and now I have some good days and bad days.

I feel it's partly due to the drugs but mostly to the Lord.

The nurses in the offices were all standing as we left, just staring at us. I was in a state of shock.

My husband kept saying, 'I'm so sorry.' He was crying and sobbing 'No' over and over again. I could hardly breathe. I felt like I was going to die right then. My husband started praying, 'Jesus please let it be me and not her.' The hardest part was watching his reaction.

We drove right to our church from the doctor's office. It was close to an hour away. We spent two or three hours with our pastor. Joe, my husband, said, 'We just found out that Karri is HIV-positive.' The pastor was so stunned he didn't know what to say. I don't think it registered with him right away.

That first night was horrific. I was really sick, vomiting, diarrhea, and the worst headache I had ever had. Joe was beside himself. We had a couple of friends come over and try to help. At that point I thought I was going to be dead by 10 P.M.—midnight for sure.

One of my girlfriends who had come by worked with the Catholic Church buddy program. She put me in touch with an HIV-positive support group.

I spoke to the man that ran the group. He told me about the support group and said I should come. This was within 24 hours of us finding out. Joe and I didn't know what to expect. We decided to go because we didn't know what else to do. Both my children had to be tested as well as Joe.

As soon as I got in the door I started crying. I just couldn't stop. A woman came over to me and asked if I wanted to come outside and talk. I went with her and we talked for a few minutes. I found we had things in common beside the HIV. We were both Christians. Since then we have become very good friends.

The first few times I went to the support group, I couldn't speak. The group was 80 percent gay men. I felt we were all in the same boat but these men had

been involved with HIV for a long time. I was the only one experiencing the shock of just finding out. Finally I decided to talk. I told a quick story of how I found out I was infected, about my two small babies. One of the guys said, 'Listen Karri, you're going to have to learn to live with this or die with this. It's your choice.'

I was scared. I felt very hopeless. I knew that I had been infected for a long time. When my T-cell count came back, it was 30. My doctor said that I'd probably been infected for eight-to-ten years. The most upsetting thing was my babies. My babies were not going to know who their mom was. They were so little and so dependent on me.

My husband and my babies were tested right after I found out. It took almost two weeks to get the results. It was the worst two weeks in my life. When the results came in, we went to the doctor's office. He came in and sat down. He said Joe is negative and Colleen, our four-year-old daughter, is negative. But Jack has shown some positive antibodies. We were kind of prepared, but it was hard to swallow. We had read that all kids under 18 months should have a PCR test. They had not done this type of test so we had to wait another

ten days of hell. The PCR test came back negative. I was elated. I had him make a copy of that test just so I could look at it over and over to be reassured my son was okay.

This all happened this past June 1996. I'm doing better now. The first month was a struggle not just emotionally; but I was also sick. I don't know when it happened but sometime after the first month I felt a sense of peace came over me. We had so many people praying for us through our church. I thought about that statement the gentleman made at the group. I decided I was going to choose to live with this thing.

We are very dedicated Christians.

I think the Lord had answered prayers for us. Before I had been diagnosed I had prayed consistently. I was so thankful for my salvation I asked the Lord regularly that He use me as a vessel to do His will. I never knew that this is how He would be using me. I believe that God can take any situation no matter how tragic it sounds and work it for the good. That is what I believe has happened in my life. It has been difficult, especially in the beginning.

Our pastor asked if he could tell the elders of the church and some of the staff who saw us come in crying that day. We didn't hear anything from them for a while. I think that they didn't know how to react. They had never been in contact with anyone with AIDS. I had spoken to the pastor when we were going through the tests on Jack. He asked how I would feel about keeping Jack out of the nursery till I got the test results on him. I was stunned. I could not believe what he said to me. It was 1996—I thought everyone at least knew the basics about transmission. I was very cold and just said, 'Fine,' and hung up. How can they ask my son to stay out of the nursery? He is no threat to anyone.

He had gotten wind that I was so upset. He called me back and we had a heated discussion on the phone. I expressed shock that he would have made the suggestion in the first place. If anything, Jack is in more danger being exposed to the other children than they would ever be of him. Furthermore, you don't know how many children are HIV-positive in that nursery right now. I was furious. He later called back humble and apologetic. He called an HIV specialist to come

to the elders meeting. They were given an HIV education session. He apologized for saying what he did and he admitted that they had been ignorant. He told me he loved me and we could bring Jack back in. Since that time our church has been very supportive both emotionally and financially.

My health has improved. I feel a lot

better. Before I had bad days and really, really bad days; and now I have some good days and bad days. I feel it's partly due to the drugs but mostly to the Lord.

We have not had sex since my diagnosis. It has been seven months. We are both hesitant. We both heard that condoms are not one hundred percent safe. I'm nervous about him becoming infected. The thing that is surprising is that he never used condoms before we found out, and we have been together for seven years. I think the more we learn, there will be a time when we will become more comfortable being sexually active. We are very affectionate. Hugging, kissing, and stroking can be fulfilling. And besides, we had a lot to deal with in the last six months. Sex is not a priority for us right now.

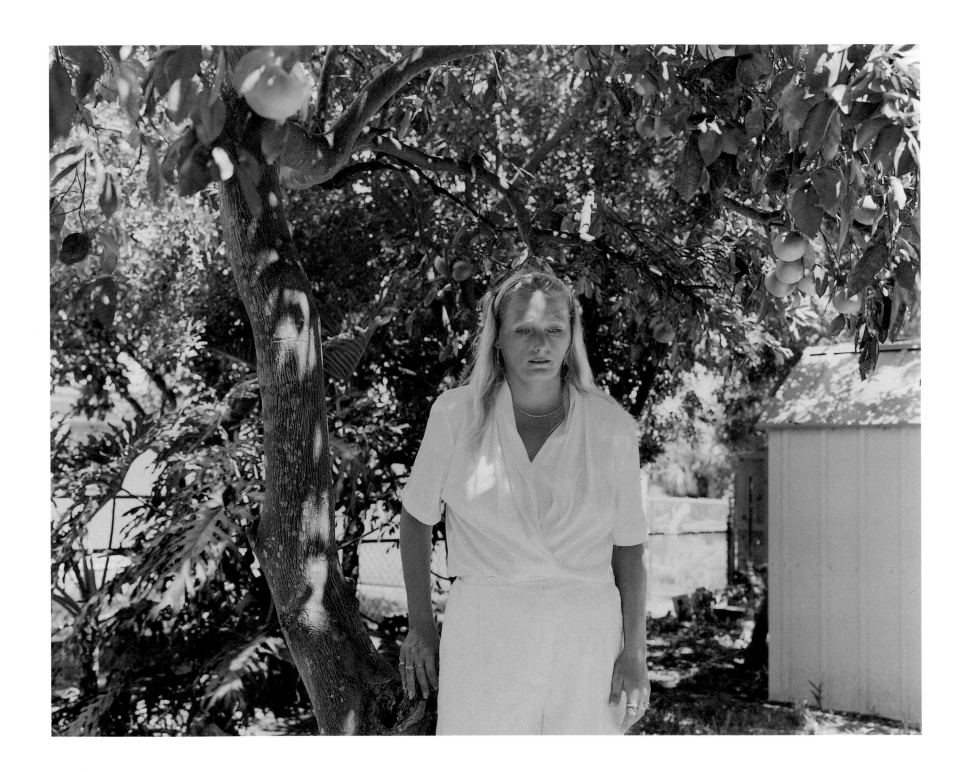

joy

37, diagnosed HIV-positive in 1994,
infected in the eighties, unsure of transmission

I was starting to get sick: fatigue and depression mostly. A couple of people took me to a church. I found spiritual release there: having God in my life and a place to feel peace. This church was doing a drive to get people tested. I decided it was time for me to find out. There was no apparent reason for me to be so sick all the time. I went to be tested because I was in all the high-risk categories. I had lots of transfusions, did drugs, and had unprotected sex. It had been on my mind for awhile.

The health department called me. They said that I should come in to have counseling. They didn't say why, but I figured it out. I was terrified at first. I just broke down and started crying. They gave me tissues and that's about it. I didn't feel like they had too much compassion. They referred me to People of Color AIDS Coalition.

Those people were very understanding. They referred me to some support groups. That really helped.

I have a relationship now with a man that loves me very much. He is a real sweetheart. He takes good care of me. He is HIV-negative. Neither of us knew I was positive when he was first attracted to me. When I found out, he was the first person that I told. He said, 'So, it's okay, I still love you and want you.'

We have a good sex life. He won't use a condom. I tried and tried, and he won't wear one. I feel guilty about this. He gives blood every month. He is a blue blood. He doesn't think I can infect him.

Most of the time I just wish it was over. I'm tired of living—like I lived too much in too short of a time. I feel really numb. I think things would be different if I wasn't sick all the time. I have two dogs. I love my dog Herby, he's Maltese. He's my sweet boy. I think I stay around just for him.

I was adopted and raised by a white couple. I always felt that my spirit belonged someplace else. I came to New Mexico in 1990 in search of my roots. I wanted to find out more about my people. I came here to Linda's house.

Linda's son, Daniel, was half Indian and half Hispanic. He understood the language of the native culture. We started hanging out. We were playing around. We didn't know what we wanted. Then I got pregnant and everything changed.

I always knew I would be a young mom. I felt ready for it, but Daniel had another view. He didn't want to work or find a job. He struggled with the responsibilities of being a dad at such a young age.

James was conceived on Mother's Day and born on January 31, 1992. Shortly after he was born, we started fighting a lot. I was nagging for him to be a better provider. We started to get violent with each other. I felt like I was going to get physically injured, so I left. Daniel's mom was protective of Daniel. She said there was no need to get a restraining order; we could pray. But I felt he needed more than prayer—he needs the justice system. It made us both very unhappy.

I checked into the psychiatric ward for depression. I felt okay there. There was a man, Jeff, who was also just breaking up. He was thirty-nine, Native American, strikingly handsome, and depressed like me. We talked a lot. I left before he did but we stayed in touch.

When I got out, Daniel wanted to get back together. I said, 'no.' He was violent. Jeff happened to stop by and asked what happened. I was bruised. He said, 'I'm getting you out of here.' He became my knight in shining armor.

He helped me go back to school. He made me feel secure, safe, and loved. Before we became intimately

shana tenendah

25, HIV-positive since January 1993, diagnosed on April 22, 1994, infected through sex

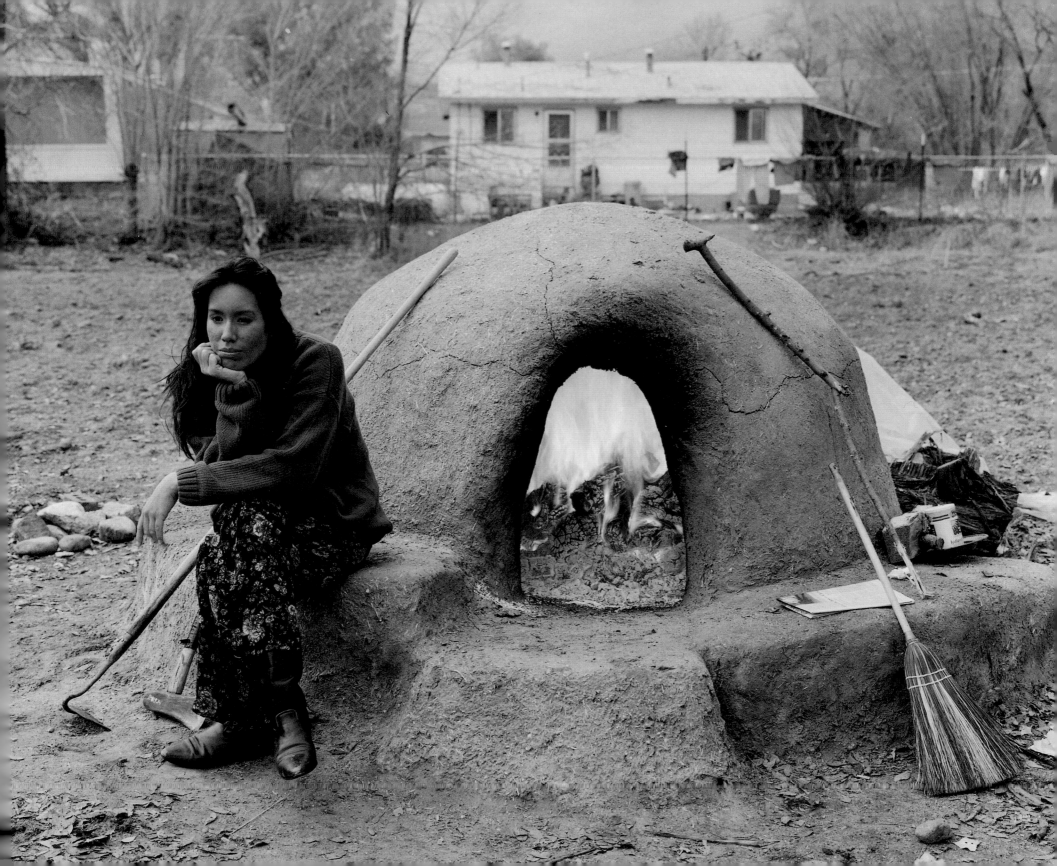

involved, I asked him, 'Is there any reason we need to use condoms?' Did he have any sexually transmitted diseases or HIV? He said, 'No, I've been tested and I'm negative.' I asked because he said in the hospital that he had a terminal illness and he wouldn't say what it was. He now told me it was lupus, and he had a bout with lung cancer. I had no reason to question him. I trusted him.

It was really wonderful. I went to college. He always wanted to help me. I went through three semesters at school before I noticed that he had a problem with alcohol. He drank every day—not to the point of being ugly or abusive, but it pushed some buttons for me.

My father is a successful, recognized doctor, but he is also an alcoholic. The lies in my family were significant. I was repeating a pattern. I was not going to do this. It was hard enough growing up in an alcoholic family. I wouldn't put my son through the same thing.

I tried every approach to get Jeff to stop. I thought I had made a good choice but I knew that I couldn't deal with the alcohol, so I asked him to leave. He was upset. He felt I had only used him to get on my feet. He wanted to get married and have children.

The last day was ugly. He called me names. I called him names. He got violent. At the end of the argument he said,

'Well guess what, I got AIDS and now so do you. You might as well stay with me because who else will want to be with you.' I remember thinking, 'Where on earth did that come from?' I just said something smart back and asked him to leave.

A few weeks later I was talking with a friend about my breakup. She had one thing to say, 'If someone told you they have AIDS, you should be tested.' I thought he was just threatening, trying to get reaction out of me.

I was nervous and scared. I was dealing with so much. I was 22, and James had just turned two.

It took me a couple more weeks before I went to get tested. April 22 the results came back. I will never forget that day. The school nurse told me to sit down. She showed me the results on paper. I started crying and didn't stop for three weeks. I felt everything—rage, numbness, betrayal, sadness, confusion, scared. More often than not, rage and numbness. That day I still had to go home and cook dinner for James.

I called my mom and she came out the next day. My first T-cell count was 189; I had an AIDS diagnosis. It takes most people years to get that low. I was scared. I was given the average two-to-five year life sentence. Then they told me that I had to test my son. For a good half a year that I was with Jeff, I had been nursing James. That was the worst three days of my life. It put me beyond rage. If he had infected my son because of whatever mental illness he had, I would kill him.

The process was so scary for him. They poked him in the toe and he screamed when they took the blood. He didn't understand what was going on. That left an imprint on my soul. They rushed the results. Until I found out, I couldn't sleep or eat. I couldn't do anything but cry and pray, and I didn't feel like it was enough.

James's test came back negative. I felt a huge relief. I had made a promise: if my son was spared, I will deal with this.

James and I spent a lot of time outside that summer. One day we were sitting in these pools of water from a river bed. It was really hot. We were splashing, having a good time. In the middle of this I realized that having AIDS can be okay. I don't like how I was infected, but there's something to be learned from it. I didn't want to be afraid anymore. I was always so afraid, afraid of everything. A lot of people hate this virus. I'm not going to do that. I started talking to my virus. I told it that I will welcome it to my body. It came unannounced, but this is my body and we need an agreement: 'You will not replicate and take over my body. I will find a way for you to get out. I won't take drugs that will kill you. I will try to live in unison with you. If you try to kill me, you will kill yourself.' I had to change my diet, quit smoking, change stress, and listen to my whole body.

When I'm not taking care of myself, I can feel it. My body responds right away. This virus has caused me to be disciplined. I realized none of us know how long we have here. Life is about quality, not quantity. Most of us want both but there is no guarantee.

I wouldn't take AZT. I wanted to use native medicine. I wanted to find a friendly way to sing it out, breathe it out, sweat it out. It wasn't about killing or death. The last thing I wanted was to have death happening in my body. I went to native ceremonies. I was open with the elders. The elders said not all of my teachers will be humans, and this is one of them. They said, 'When you have a teacher you listen to it, respect it, and don't step in front of it. Stay close to the native medicine and you will be okay.' I stopped feeling like I was dying. I would tell friends what I was learning and they would ask, 'How long do you have left to live?'

The biggest thing HIV taught me is that if you look at our track record as human beings on this planet, it's not so good. We've damaged ourselves and we've damaged our earth. It really makes sense that at some point our mother earth would kick out a virus that is a mirror for us, give us a plague to remind us of who we are and the damage that we are capable of and also give us an invitation to change our behavior.

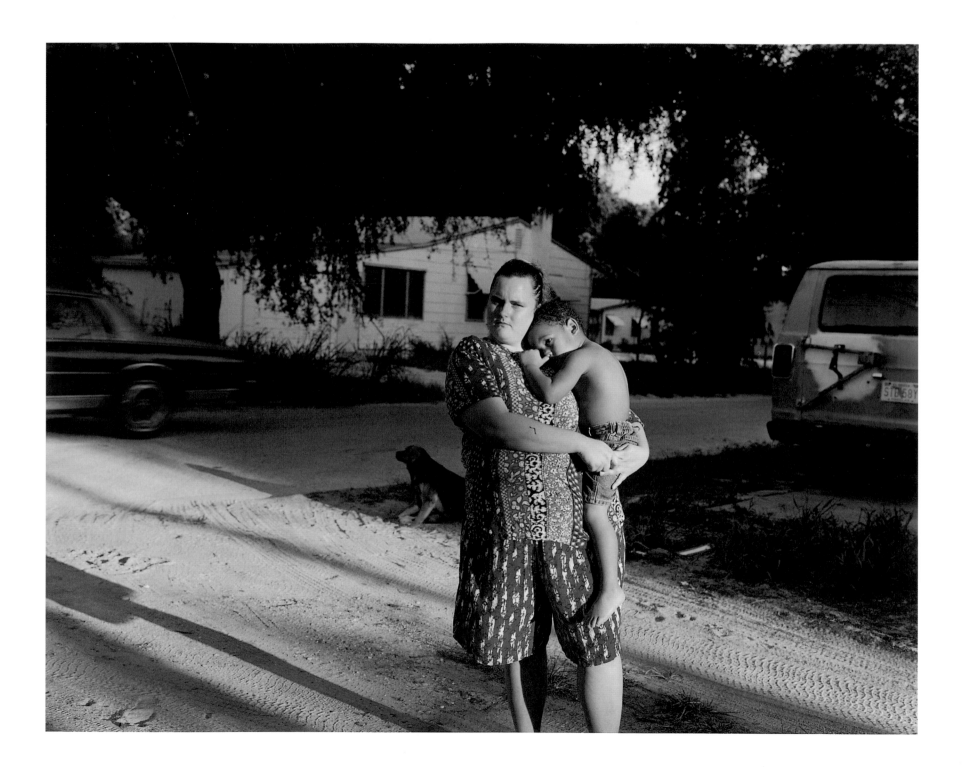

tarrilyn

26, diagnosed HIV-positive in December 1995,

infected through sex

Me and my best friend went to the Department of Health for some other tests. Someone had told her she had gonorrhea. It's an all-day process to get anything done at this place, so I figured while I'm here why don't I have the tests also. They asked us if we wanted an HIV test. We both said okay.

They sent my friend a letter telling her to come in. I didn't get any letter so I thought I was fine. I went in with her. We were joking that if we tested positive we'd get really high and jump off the La Concha building, the highest building in Key West. We wanted to go out with a big bang. I kept thinking, 'She's positive, she's positive.'

I went in first and he asked if I'd ever had an HIV test before. I said, 'Yes, it was negative.' He told me I had a positive result. I went into shock. I was crying. I threw myself against the wall. The doctor said, 'You can take medicines and live a healthy life.' He started telling me about other people, that HIV made them better persons. I didn't want to hear any of this.

He then gave my best friend her results as I was standing there. She was negative. She was holding on to me. I had to get out of there. He gave me a whole file of information. I ran out. I gave my friend my last ten dollars so she could take a cab.

I worked at a restaurant where one of the waiter's had a partner with AIDS. I had already had a conversation with him before. I wanted to call him, but I didn't have his number. I asked my boss at work if she could give it to me. She said she couldn't, so I asked her to please call him and tell him I need to talk to him. I finally got in touch and he said I could come over. Before I left, my boss asked what's wrong. I said, 'Unless you have a cure, you can't help me.' She knew about this other man having AIDS. She hugged me and said I would be all right. I went there and talked to him for a long time. When I left there I was a lot more relieved.

I had calmed down. My next fear was if I infected the guy I was sleeping with. We used protection in the beginning but we just recently stopped.

He was working when I went in the restaurant that day. He saw how upset I was. He thought I was pregnant. He asked my boss what I had said and she told him, 'You need to talk to her.'

He came to my house and asked, 'What's wrong?' I was sitting on the couch crying. I said, 'We need to talk.' He said, 'Look, if you're pregnant it's okay.' I said, 'I wish I could tell you that I was.' He said, 'If you're not pregnant, what is it?'

I told him I was positive and he went into shock. I started consoling him—how to get tested; what the odds were of him being infected. We agreed, regardless of what will happen, we will be friends. When he left, I thought it was basically over. I was worried that he was going to hate me.

He took a long time to go get tested. He didn't come

over for three days. On the third day he came over and we had protected sex. He wanted to let me know that I was okay. Our relationship got closer. In some ways we are still close. We hadn't gotten into that boyfriend–girlfriend phase yet. We'd only been going out for a couple of months. He finally got tested a month later and it was negative. I was so relieved. I don't think I could have handled it if I knew I infected someone. That relationship ended, not because of HIV but because I found another man.

I found out December 12, 1995, but I know I have been infected longer because my T-cells were low, 388. I went through four books on HIV in a month. I believe I was infected by my son's father. In the summer of 1995, he had called me on the phone. He wanted to work things out. He was not a good man. He used to beat me, so I didn't want anything to do with him. He asked me, 'Why didn't you visit me while I was in the hospital?' I said, 'I didn't know you were in there.' He said, 'You know that medicine AZT?' I said, 'Yeah that's for people with AIDS.' He said, 'That is the medicine I'm taking.'

I hadn't tested positive at that time but that didn't alarm me because I hadn't had sex with him for six years,

Right now, I'm really happy.

I've started doing things I have never done before.

I take the kids to the park. I used

to spend time with my friends instead of the kids.

and I'd tested since then. I can only guess it was wrong, or I wasn't showing the antibodies yet because the first test came back negative. The other three people I'd been with were all negative.

I have an eight-year-old boy, Aaron, and a four-year-old, Charles—we call him CJ. When I found out that first day, I looked at my kids and I cried and cried. I talked to my older son's school. Aaron has emotionally handicapped problems. I talked to his teacher. I decided I wasn't going to tell Aaron. I told him I was sick. My mom is diabetic and I told him I was like her—I had to take medicine but I will be okay. I didn't tell him the word HIV. I didn't have them tested. I didn't think I could deal with it then. Now I figure they are healthy. When I first found out, someone told me kids don't do well with HIV.

They don't hide it as long as adults.

Right now, I'm really happy. I've started doing things I have never done before. I take the kids to the park. I used to spend time with my friends instead of the kids. The kids always came second. Now they're rarely ever away from me. Life is too short. I strongly believe you can kill yourself by breaking your own heart—just lying in bed feeling bad. I don't want to die like that. My dad died like that. He wasn't HIV-positive, but he was depressed. I don't deal with negative people anymore. All that gossip "he said–she said" stuff. I have found more peace with myself. I worry about everyone still, but I now take care of myself first. The man I'm with now, we have problems but I don't revolve my life around him like I have in the past. I see him when I see him. If my kids have someplace to go, I go there instead of hanging with my boyfriend.

I lived with a man who was HIV-positive for two years. I took an HIV test every six months. One time the test came back positive. There was slippage and breakage of condoms from not using them properly. I was never scared about being infected even when the condom would fail. Living with a man who is HIV-positive, you take it on as your own. You're living with it every day. It's almost as if you have the disease.

Most people knew that he was positive. We never hid it. After I tested positive, only my oldest daughter knew. She had come with me when I went for the results. After the nurse told me that my test came back positive, I tried to remain calm. I was in shock even though I knew that this was always a possibility. I went into the waiting room and I told my daughter. I knew that she was upset also but she handled it well. She became my support. She would say,

'Don't worry mom, you will be okay.' She was 21 years old.

I didn't choose to tell my children, it was really forced on me. It was some holiday and they were going to visit their father's family. But his family insisted that they all be tested before they come up. They knew I was positive. I was outspoken but I wanted control of who I told and when. I wasn't prepared. I felt compelled to tell them why they were all being tested. They were already educated about HIV. They were upset when I told them I was infected. They were only eight, ten, and fifteen. I gave in to having them all tested because I wanted them to be able to visit their family. I feel family is important. I could have said 'forget it,' but it wouldn't be fair. In the end it all has turned out okay. Now their father and his family are educated. They act a lot different now about HIV. They have children who have learned more about HIV than they would through TV

debbie diamond

45, diagnosed HIV-positive September 30, 1992, infected through sex

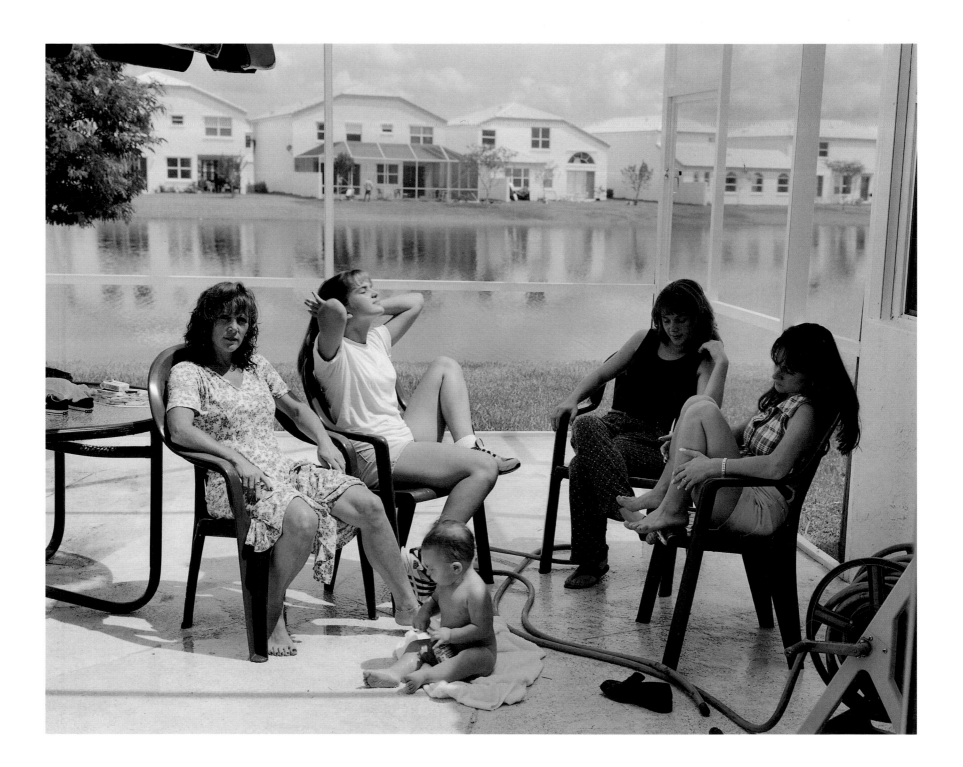

My hope is that no one else has to die from this disease.

AIDS is all over the world. . . . Too much death.

Too much pain for the sons, daughters, mothers, and fathers.

I can't comprehend why they haven't found

something that can really make this illness manageable.

or school. This makes me happy. It's like a ripple effect.

I feel wonderful right now. I'm not on any medication. My T-cells are average and my viral load is low. I do vitamins, herbs, and acupuncture. Nothing regularly. I listen to my body. If I'm under a lot of stress I do things to take care of it. I meditate, relax, and try to be happy. It's unfortunate to say this, but HIV has given me back my will to live.

My lover died two years ago July.

He was a dynamic person. Always dancing, loving. We had our fights but I loved him. I was with him up to the end

with the exception of his death. We separated a month before he died. He had become angry and bitter. He was humiliated. The doctors had given us no hope. His family came down and they took care of him. I had to leave for my own sanity. I couldn't go through his death. Just a month before, in September 1990, I had lost my son, Frankie.

Frankie had been misdiagnosed with a heart condition. He was in college and working full time. His roommate had left and it was too much for him. I suggested he come home. The day he moved in he was getting bad heart palpitations. He called his doctor and his doctor told him to put his legs up and take some medication that he had given him. We laid on the bed and were joking around. I kissed him goodnight. In the morning I found him, he was dead. I broke every window in my house. I kicked in the walls. I was never the same. Later, the autopsy would show he needed a pacemaker. I sued the doctor and won. It didn't make my son come back.

I couldn't go through it again.

I was afraid to wake up and find Bobby dead. I had to leave. I guess HIV can make you selfish. The loss would have been too much. When I think about him I remember him when he was well—a fun-loving and healthy man. I consider that a gift.

He was angry when I left. A part of him wanted me to stay, but I think a bigger part wanted me to leave. It's different when a significant other takes care of someone who is dying. It's so humiliating for a person who took such good care of himself to not be able to do the simplest things. I think I would want my children, compared to a lover or spouse, to care for me if I was dying. Lucky thing I have four children—one of them has to take me, or at least share.

My hope is that no one else has to die from this disease. AIDS is all over the world. When I attended the 11th International Conference on HIV/AIDS in Vancouver, I learned how many people are infected—are still being infected. Too much death. Too much pain for the sons, daughters, mothers, and fathers. I can't comprehend why they haven't found something that can really make this illness manageable. Because it certainly isn't the new treatments that have come out. Most people can't afford the treatments, and side effects can be debilitating. They are not for everybody but they are being prescribed to all HIV-positive people. It definitely isn't a cure. It's ridiculous. It gives false hope to the youth. They stop using condoms because, "Hey, there is a treatment now!" This is not pregnancy or the "clap"—this is their life.

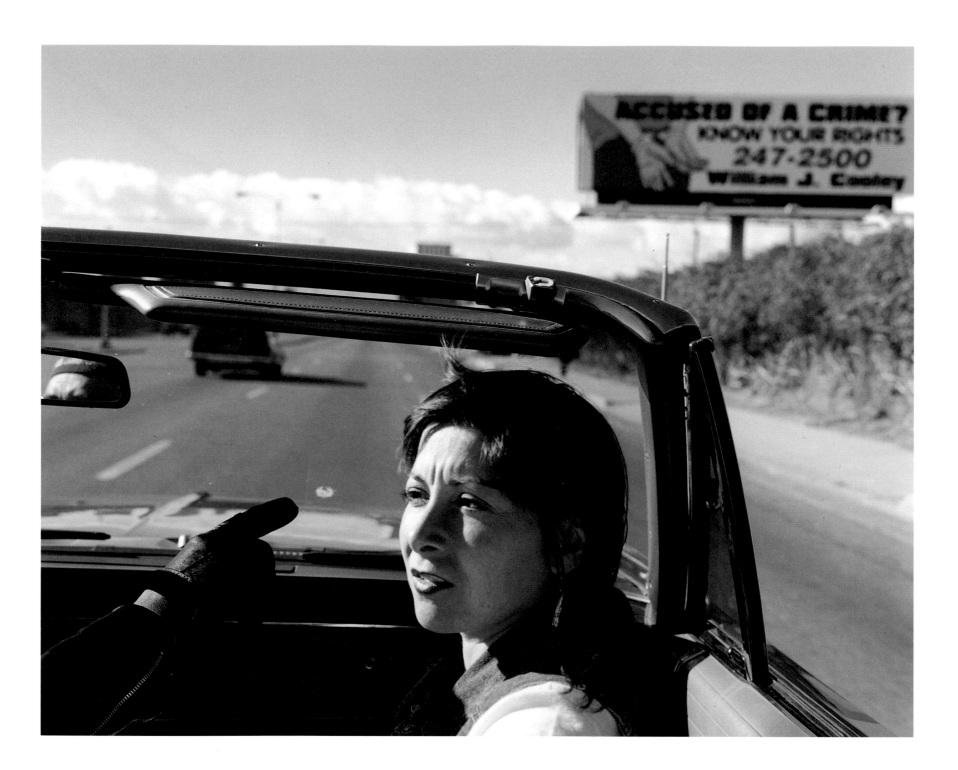

In 1983 I had the typical symptoms of seroconversion sickness: unexplained rashes all over my torso, swollen lymph glands, chills, and a fever.

Shortly after that my lymph glands became very swollen. My doctor thought I might have lymphoma or Hodgkin's. When the tests came back negative for cancer, my doctor said I was fine. For the next four years I had fatigue and strange little things. One time I had cellulitis in my ankle after ice skating. The doctor told me that only happens to old people. It dawned on me maybe I have Epstein-Barr. There was an Epstein-Barr specialist across the street from my doctor so I thought I would check him out. On the first visit he said, 'What do you think about testing for HIV? Why don't we rule that out?' I said, 'No problem.'

Immediately after I went to this new doctor he wanted me to get B$_{12}$ and magnesium shots. He was very holistic oriented. I started going every week for these shots. The second week after the physical the doctor called me into his office. Usually the nurse gives me the shots and I leave. I had completely forgotten about the HIV test. He told me that it had come back positive. He was so cool about it. He was so ahead of his time. He said even though you're HIV-positive, you're in good health and you never have to get sick. Now this was 1987, the peak of AIDS hysteria. It was an incredible thing for him to say. A month later AZT was approved and they were prescribing it like Flintstones chewables. People were popping it around the clock. My doctor was so against it. He knew it was incredibly toxic. He told me, 'There is no way I want you to start taking that.' This was an Armenian man who had a family practice of mainly immigrants from Russia.

andrea acosta

36, HIV-positive since 1983, diagnosed March 1987, infected through sex

At that time there was all these gay physicians that had become HIV specialists. They had the gay clientele. They were prescribing AZT to all their patients just because it was the only medication available to treat HIV. It had nothing to do with whether it was effective or not. They were desperate. My humble family-practice guy knew more than any of them. He intrinsically knew that the best thing was to treat my immune system holistically. There wasn't any urgency to prescribe drugs.

He was great. I went to him for eight years once a week and got my B_{12}, magnesium, and folic acids shots. Every time I saw him he would tell me I was doing great. My lymph glands went down completely.

The only time that my T-cells dropped was after a catastrophic earthquake. I was in Los Angeles. When the earthquake hit I was living about a mile from the epicenter. There where aftershocks every day. You could never relax—you were always waiting for the next blast. That showed me more than anything how stress affects the immune system. It was the first time my T-cells had gone under 500.

My T-cells had been in the 200's since the earthquake. I moved to Albuquerque and have been here for three years now. I just had a T-cell count done and they were over 500.

My viral load went from 25,000 to 8,000 in one year. This is with no western medications. I only do holistic therapies, besides my beloved Prozac.

The greatest impact the virus has had on my life is concerning relationships. I always had a "jerk magnet." A "jerk magnet" is an internal device to which people who are jerks, mainly of the co-dependent variety, are attracted. Through electrical currents in the air or just behavior patterns imprinted since a small child, said magnet tends to draw partners who are of a parasitic nature—otherwise known as "jerks." I was living with a guy for a year who I didn't know was a jerk. It definitely emerged when I found out I was positive. One thing about HIV—it is a true litmus test of whether friends, family, or partners are jerks.

Fortunately, through a lot of therapy and self-help books, I learned to let go of my jerk magnet and consequently I met a great guy. We met on a movie location in Hollywood. I'm not going into it, but we fell in love, got married, and moved to Albuquerque.

Since we moved here I have run a statewide HIV Speakers Bureau. It's important being able to go public. In Los

I was living with a guy for a year who I didn't know was a jerk.
It definitely emerged when I found out I was positive.
One thing about HIV—it is a true litmus test of whether friends,
family, or partners are jerks.

Angeles I went on talk shows. I wore these floozy wigs. They always gave me platinum blonde Marilyn Monroe numbers. I wore dark glasses; hid behind screens. I never quite went as far as having my voice altered. I guess I should have because everyone knew it was me anyway. After Geraldo, some guy I hadn't seen in years showed up at my apartment and said, 'Weren't you just on Geraldo?'

I'm the first of two women in the San Francisco Cohert Long Term Non-Progressor Study. I had to wait a year because it was closed to women. It started as a gay man health study in which they were looking at hepatitis in gay men. After the HIV test was available in 1985, they went as far back as '78 and tested for HIV. The study evolved into looking at how some people in the group were progressing or not. They noticed a percentage of HIV-positive men who were not progressing at all. There are several people who have been infected at least since 1978 and have no signs of immune suppression.

I'm a slow progressor because my T-cells went down, even though they have gone up again. I have never been sick, so I tried to get over the T-cell game and focus on my good health.

I will always thank Dr. Tilkian. I largely attribute my health to his powerful words and his belief in my ability to stay healthy. It's more than just luck. I work really hard in a multitude of ways, including vitamins, herbs, nutrition, positive attitude, exercise, and changing my life if it becomes too stressful. The natural thing to do when you find out you're HIV-positive is to freak out and believe it's a death sentence. I mean, that is what the whole world is saying. I'm glad I had a rebellious nature, was blessed with a great doctor, and had lots of therapy.

kristine

29, HIV-positive since January 1989, infected through sex

I know exactly how long I have been infected—since January 1989. When I was infected my body freaked out, my glands were huge, and I had rashes. The classic seroconversion sickness. I was bewildered. I had never been sick. I went to the doctor. He gave me some cream and sent me home. I found out later I had shingles, which is a classic sign of HIV. It went away and everything was fine. The doctor never suggested I should be tested. Why should he? I was living in Chicago and going to school. I didn't sleep with that many people. I was a normal college girl living a normal college life. I guess I just got unlucky loving the wrong person. I never had contact again with the man who infected me. We dated, things didn't work out, life went on.

I had been married for six months. I was basically a newlywed. We talked about HIV because his brother had AIDS. I asked, 'Have you been tested?' He said, 'Yes.' So I thought I should take a test. When I went for the results, the nurse practitioner tried to make small talk. I felt that she was nervous. Finally, she said, 'Your test came back positive.' It was the end and the beginning of everything.

She went into the thing that there is hope, blah blah blah. I walked out of the waiting room. I walked right past my husband and I said, 'I have it.' He just followed me out. We dealt with it by making jokes almost right away. He opened the door for me and said 'AIDS before beauty.' We became hysterical. I eventually shut down for probably two or three years.

I did my vitamins and read the AIDS newsletters, but that was it. I felt as if there was no one out there I could relate to. It made me feel like a pariah. I would just lie in my bed and cry. I was 23 and I was faced with my own mortality. I kept thinking I would be dead in year: 'I'm toast, I'm gone.

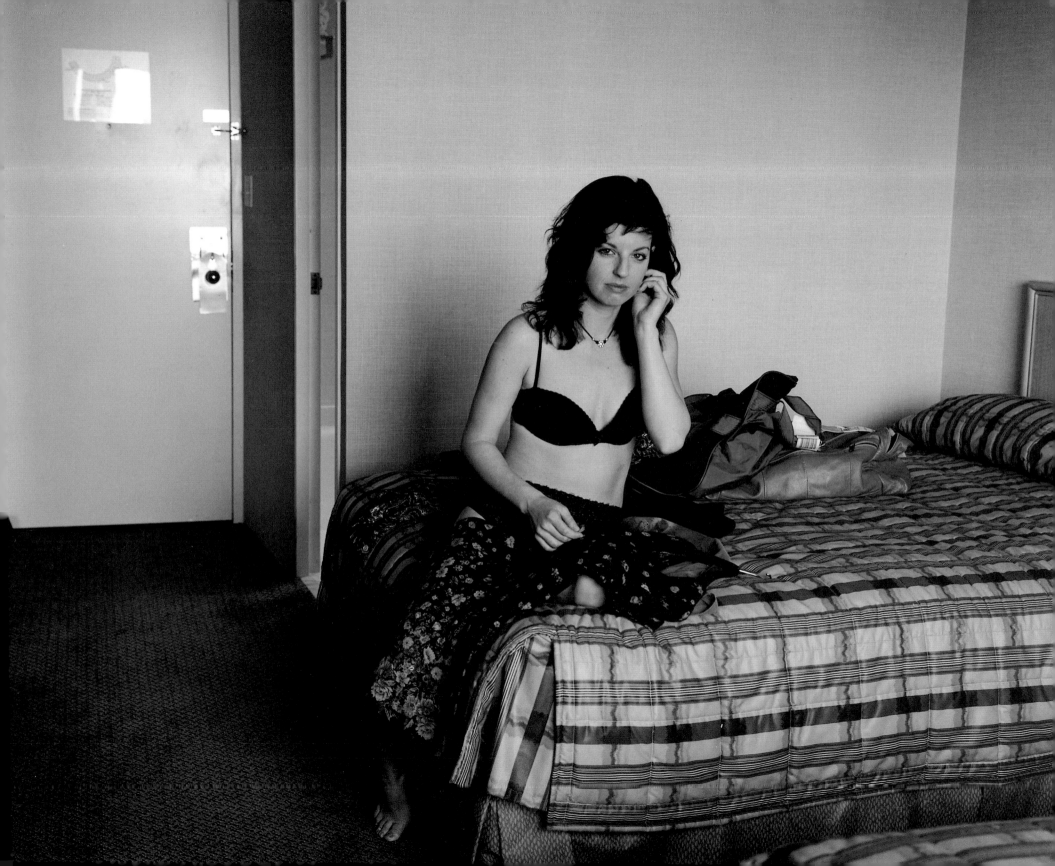

I wanted to use a condom

with the man that infected me. . . . I remember he said,

'I won't get you pregnant, baby. I will pull out.'

Well, that was true, he didn't get me pregnant—

he pulled out, but he did infect me.

I might as well go out back and dig my grave.'

They put me on AZT. Then I really felt bad. I had headaches, nausea, fatigue. Before the AZT I felt okay. The first doctor I went to was horrible. She asked me when I thought I was infected. I told her I knew exactly when I was infected. She acted as if there was no way I would be able to know such a thing. She made me feel as if I was a really bad person and did bad things. I was unlucky. I could have won the lotto; I could have gotten HIV. I got HIV.

My marriage was doomed to begin with. I think it lasted longer because of HIV. He had medical insurance. There was a little bit of guilt on his side and insecurity on mine. Eventually I had a nervous breakdown and then I really

shut down. We separated while he was working in Malaysia. I moved in with my grandmother and hid out all the time. When he came back we tried to get back together. It lasted for about a year; it didn't work. I decided I wasn't dead. It had been five years and I was still here. I wasn't going to let it take one more day from me. I needed to start living. I finally said to him, 'Let's get a divorce.' I always say the marriage didn't end because of HIV, it ended because he was an asshole.

I moved to Seattle. I'd never been there but I thought it would be a cool place to be. It was the best decision I ever made in my life. I go to school and work, I have friends. I go hiking, there's the ocean. It's all so beautiful here. It's definitely better than sitting in a little room waiting to die.

None of my friends know about my infection. I feel eventually they will know. I don't want to be the Northwest AIDS Poster Child. I'm involved in a lot of AIDS organizations. But I want people to know me, not me as a disease.

My grandmother tries to brush it over. She is always saying, 'Doesn't she look healthy? She looks so good!' In the meantime I'm walking around with a tattered immune system. There's been some bumps, but in general my family has been good. They try really hard.

I would not know that I had this disease unless I had been tested. I get rashes and swollen glands, but other than that there is nothing to indicate that I have AIDS or HIV. Sometimes I think about how many other women are infected and don't even know. Sometimes I wonder if it would be better if I didn't know. When I start thinking like that I remember that if I didn't know, I would be putting other people at risk. I think it's important to be tested so you can protect the ones you love. I wouldn't want to hurt someone I love.

I wanted to use a condom with the man that infected me. We were only together a couple of times. I didn't have enough self-esteem. I remember he said, 'I won't get you pregnant, baby. I will pull out.' Well, that was true, he didn't get me pregnant—he pulled out, but he did infect me.

I will not tell you that my life is so much better because of HIV. Believe me, I would be much happier without it. I might look at things deeper now, but I would be happier to be shallow and not have it.

Sometimes I don't even want to think about it anymore. I might be in denial but I'm not sick. I feel fabulous and I look good.

I have a lot of trepidation about the picture and book. I'm shot in my undies. There's so much misconception about HIV girls being bad, and here I'm in my undies. I talked to my mom about it and she said that as long as it's a nice picture then it's all right. The truth is, no matter what I say or look like, some people will think bad things about me. There is nothing I can do about it.

I think I live in a state of numb terror. I'm just scared witless but I don't let myself access it.

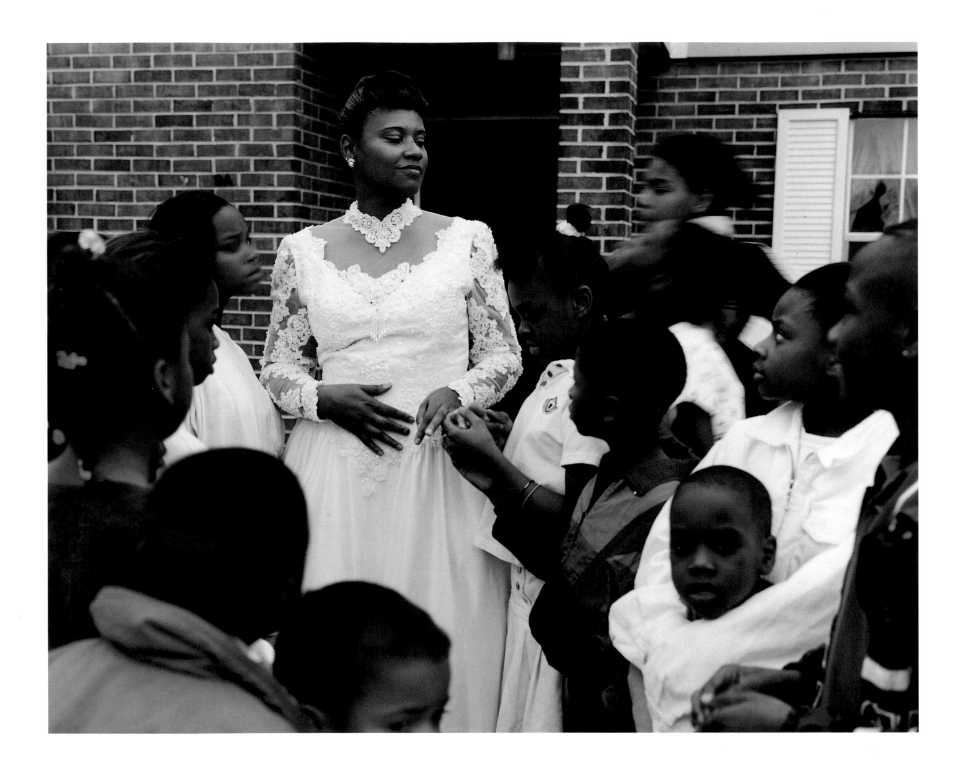

I know who infected me. He called for me to come see him in the hospital. I knew what he was going to tell me. I had to pray before I went there for the strength to not be angry—that I could just be there for him. He was real sick. They thought he was going to die. His lungs had collapsed. I knew this might be my last opportunity to have closure with him.

I didn't say nothing. I let him talk. He said he was sorry and he wondered how many people's lives he messed up. He was using drugs when we were together. I don't know if he knew he was infected when he was with me. At this point it really doesn't matter. I don't hold him responsible because I chose not to use condoms. I never used condoms till I knew I was infected.

I thought I picked my men well. He was one of the only men I dated who used IV drugs. I had vaguely heard of AIDS. I was using then. It was not anything that would affect me. I never had any sexually transmitted diseases. In 1989, I got clean.

My drug was cocaine. I never shot it up. I never had a record, not even a traffic ticket. One day I was in the wrong place. I was arrested. But what really made me change my life was when my oldest daughter said she was tired of hurting. She said, 'Why don't you just take a gun and put it to your head and kill yourself?' When I had my kids, it was no accident I had them because I wanted them. I thought about losing them and that was it. I knew it was time for help. I went into treatment the next day.

Some friends of mine who were in recovery would get tested every year. When they would talk about it I would say, 'Oh yeah I've been tested.' I'd never been tested. Why was I saying I have been? So I made a decision to get tested.

tracie edness-etheredge

38, HIV-positive since 1989, diagnosed in 1991,

infected through sex

I never thought it would really be positive.

My oldest daughter went with me. I remember before I left the house to get the results I said, 'God, let your presence be there before I get there.' My daughter asked, 'Why are you saying that?' I said, 'I just need His presence there.' When they gave me the results I fainted. When they brought me to, I was crying. I asked to have some time to myself. I cried and prayed. I felt hopeless and devastated. When I could get myself together, I went and got my daughter. We went to the car. I wouldn't talk. I went in my room and started crying. My daughter came in to say she loved me and then we cried.

I went into a deep depression for about six months. At that time I became suicidal—I just didn't know which way I wanted to do it. Amidst this journey, I ran into this man. He kept following me. I cussed him out but he kept following me wherever I went. Finally I was so depressed. I asked him if I could talk to him. We sat on a curb, I shared about my diagnosis and what I was thinking of doing. In return, he told me he was positive and had been living with it for five years. I didn't know if I should believe him or not. He took my number and gave me his card. He called about twice a week. He would say I need to get

involved in a support group. I finally went to Out Reach, Inc. Eventually I became a volunteer.

He might have known I was positive because I would go to this clinic where all the AIDS patients were. I would look at these very sick people to help me have the strength to kill myself. I believe he might have seen me up there. He never told me. Now I think that he was a guardian angel—to give me hope and get me connected.

My biggest fear was no one would want me. I didn't want my kids to suffer. I thought I would be dead in six months.

I started getting educated. I went to this doctor. He would sit and educate me about the differences between HIV and AIDS. I started to feel like I could live with this thing.

The first relationship with someone not infected was with a woman. It was inspired because I didn't think anyone would want me, and she accepted me as I was, HIV and all. This person was my friend. She was there for me. She treated me nice. It eventually became real crazy. I don't know what happened. I was not sure I wanted to live a gay lifestyle. This women was definitely gay, and I was ambivalent.

The relationship became abusive—physically and verbally. We both ended up abusing each other. I was secretive about the virus. Only my daughter and past lovers knew. I forbade her to talk with anyone about it. The pressure just built up. A lot had to do with me talking about being married. All my life I knew I wanted to be married. She knew when I talked about this that I meant being married to a man. She would throw it up about me being positive. That was painful. It became physical. We ended the relationship. Now we are very good friends. I feel in my heart that if something happened she would be there for me.

Then I became involved with Ben. I needed someone and he was there. I ended up having a lot of good feelings for him. We were dating, but he was in early recovery. I thought it best that we end it so he could have a chance to get clean.

I was in another unsuccessful relationship, then Ben came back into my life. We dated for awhile and then we stopped seeing each other. I dated other men but it seemed that it always came back to Ben.

I had to ask, 'Why does God keep bringing us together?' I knew I loved him. He was such a sweet person—I just didn't know if I could give the love back that he gave me.

He asked me to marry him. I told him I needed to pray on it. God said it was okay. I went and I told him that evening that I would marry him. He wanted to do a fall or spring wedding. He felt those times were about new beginnings. I didn't want to wait because we might change our minds. I picked October 19, my birthday.

We had a beautiful wedding, but on our honeymoon I lost it. When he pulled out the condoms and put them on the dresser I just burst out in tears. He held me and told me it was going to be okay. It just hit me so hard that I have this virus. Here I'm married and I can never have unprotected sex with my husband. This was supposed to be the time to share precious and intimate feelings. Deep down inside I know that condoms don't take away from those feelings. You can still love intimately. I had to go through it and I might go through it again. Sometimes it doesn't feel real good inside—just every now and again. I try not to dwell on it. Condoms don't stop anything really, except body fluids.

It's only been three months. We are going through some changes right now, but I wouldn't give it up for anything. We are both used to living by ourselves and we have to adjust to some things. There're a lot of things we need to learn about living together. Now it's some test. But I'm glad I got married. He is my husband and I love him.

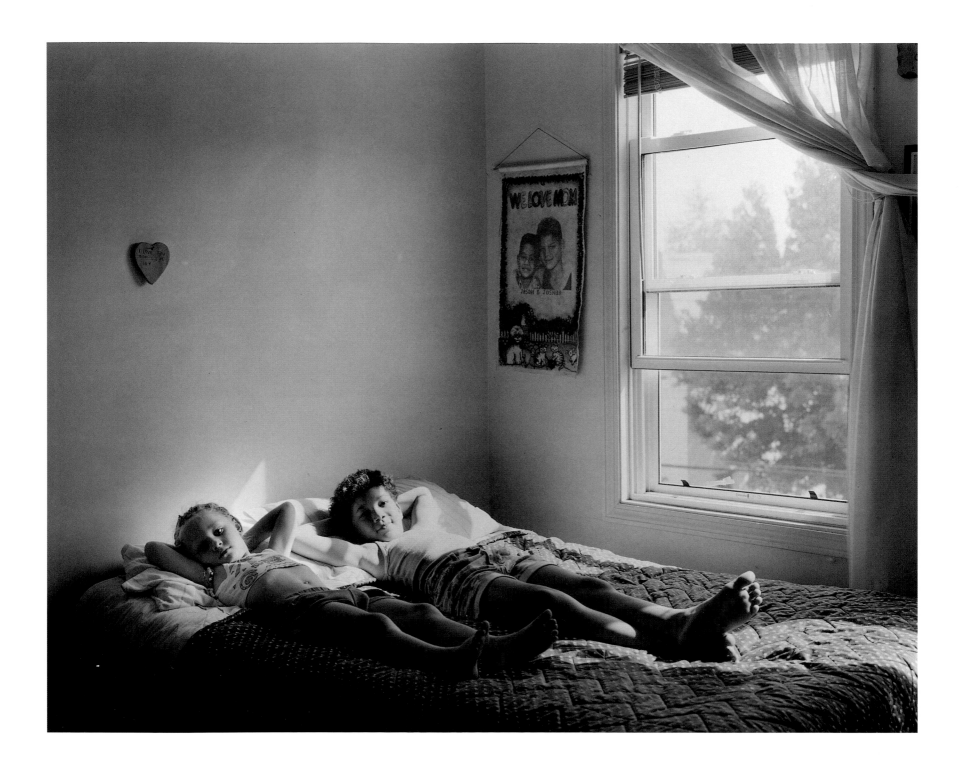

I trusted this guy so much. I knew him for a long time. Well, things happen. He knew that he was HIV-positive when he infected me. His wife died from AIDS. I kept asking, 'Are you okay? Have you been to the doctor?' He said yes, that he was okay.

I went to take HIV/AIDS training because my sister died from AIDS. I wanted to make a difference in someone's life because I couldn't be there for my sister. I found out she was sick about a week before she died. I went to see her in the hospital. Her doctor called me and said she was in a coma and I should come. Later he told me she had AIDS. I felt great pain. It hurt so bad just to see her laying there and knowing I couldn't do anything. It was the hardest thing to see my sister like that. She was my only sister. I don't think she told anyone what she had been going through.

At about the same time as the HIV training, I went for a physical. I asked if he would give me an HIV test. I did it on my own. I figured it's something that everyone should do. Two weeks later the results came back positive. I was afraid to talk to anyone. I heard so many things—how people walk away, how they treat you.

I have four boys and two granddaughters that I take care of. My grandchildren are only six and nine. I was even thinking of killing myself. I figured I would die and they would suffer. Fortunately, I began to get educated about HIV.

I don't go to support groups because I have to deal with this myself. I have people who help and I have a counselor that comes to my house once a week. I like to keep things private. I stay with my kids. All I have is my kids. They are my life.

I get afraid. This is a borrowed life. Everyone gets afraid that something will happen. I accept it the way it is.

adriana rivera

48, diagnosed HIV-positive in 1994, infected through sex

patsy stewart

43, HIV-positive since 1988, diagnosed in April 1993, infected through sex

I went to the doctor for an exam.

She took eight tubes of blood. As a joke, I said 'You're taking so much blood why don't you take an HIV test?' She told me, 'There is no need for you to take that test. You're not in a risk category.'

I don't know why I said it. I didn't know anything about AIDS. It didn't affect me. They always portrayed it as a gay disease. Heterosexual women didn't get it.

The first test they lost. That's when I thought there was something going on. They sent me directly to the lab the second time. When I went for my results, my doctor sent another doctor in to tell me. I don't know if she was embarrassed because she didn't want me to take the test in the first place, or what. We sat down and he said, 'I have some bad news . . . you tested positive for the virus.' I thought I was going to die: 'This is it.' I didn't know anything about HIV.

The doctor was very standoffish. I sat there in shock. He said, 'Do you have any questions?' I couldn't think, all I wanted to do was leave. I came home and I immediately took a plate, silverware, and a cup and put them separate—I didn't know anything about transmission. My youngest boy, Kenny, was still at home. I wanted to do what I could to make sure he didn't get infected. I even set aside a bar of soap.

I was too scared to tell my son. I didn't know how to tell him. I called my best friend, Gary, and told him. He came over and we just sat and cried. When I finally got the courage to tell Kenny, Gary came over to be with me. Kenny was a senior in high school. He was getting ready for the prom and graduation night, and here I was going to have to blow his senior year. I couldn't hide it. I had never lied to him. I felt I was deceiving him for the two weeks it took me to tell him.

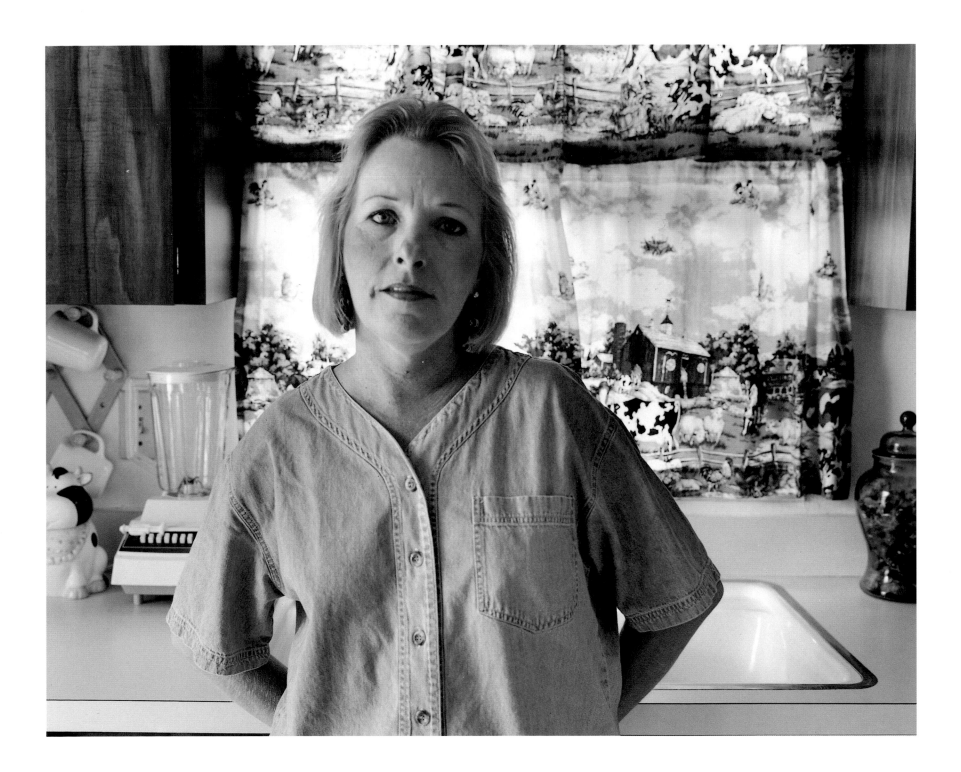

I told him and he was mad. In fact, he voiced he wished he could find the person he thought infected me so he could kill him.

I don't blame anyone.

It was my own responsibility. I should have used protection, even though at the time I was infected there was no talk of women getting AIDS. We were the silent population becoming infected. That makes me mad. I think they should have targeted regular programming on TV. Even now they don't do enough. It's always younger people—never people 35 and up. People my age don't feel they have anything to worry about.

I went to the mall to get some information about HIV. They had no books at all on AIDS. I found three books at a small independent book store downtown. I went to a support group. The more I learned, the more I felt assured I was going to be okay. After about six months of being on the pity pot—'why me, boohoo'—I decided to do volunteer work. Volunteering made me a much stronger person.

I have dated positive guys. One man recently passed away. I met him at Suncoast AIDS Network. We went out a couple of times but it didn't work out. We remained friends after we split. I would joke with him and say he needed a "yes-dear, whatever-you-say-dear" type of woman, and I'm far from that.

It was hard when he died. It was a slap of reality. I have only been to three services since I have become involved in the HIV community because it's a very difficult thing for me to do.

I have had ups and downs. I had PCP. I also had a hysterectomy. I had cysts and constant bleeding. They didn't know if it was HIV-related. There has been no Ob-gyn that deals with HIV women in this area. All the positive women I know have gynecological problems and none of the doctors really understand the connection to HIV.

When I started to have problems I went to see a doctor. I told him I was positive and he put this big, red sticker on my chart saying I was positive. I was lying in the stirrups when he came in. He said, 'Remind us when you come in to tell us that you're positive so we can take extra precautions.' I said, 'What!' He said, 'Yes, so we can put hazardous material in a proper container.' After the exam he walks out. The nurse comes in and tells me I can get dressed. Then she told me to take the paper off the table and put my gown in a hazard bag.

I dressed and left my gown and the table paper right where they were. The doctor hands me a prescription and says, 'I will need to see you in three months.' I told him, 'I will never step foot in your door again, and I will make sure every HIV caseworker in Pinellas county knows how ignorant you are so no woman will ever have to be insulted by you.' And that is what I did.

I wasn't feeling good as it was—how dare this man treat me like this! I'm not less than anyone because I have HIV. That is the day I really became strong and realized I wasn't taking anyone's shit. You don't have choices on Medicaid. They make you feel this is who you have to go see. But that's not so. I don't deserve to be treated like a second-class citizen. I worked hard all my life.

I used to work in auto parts for 17 years. I started out in 1970. I went to vocational school for auto mechanics. I had to fight to get in. I had just bought a '55 Chevy circle track racer. I didn't know a spark plug from an oil filter. I really wanted to learn. Then I got pregnant. They wouldn't let me do anything at school because I was pregnant, so I switched to a more conventional field for a woman: business education. I hated it! I thought if I couldn't be an auto mechanic I could do the next best thing: sell parts. I started out as a cashier and in six months I was a manager. I loved my work.

I finally had to stop working. I was the manager of an auto-parts store. I worked ten hours a day, six days a week. All I could do was work, come home, eat, and go to bed. My T-cells went down every month. Quitting work was one of the hardest decisions I ever made.

I speak a lot at high schools. Everyone stereotypes people with AIDS. They say 'You did that, you deserve it.' It makes an impact on kids that I'm a mother and grandmother.

Last week I was at Curlies. My girlfriend is a bartender there. She says, 'I want you to meet this guy.' I had one of my AIDS T-shirts on. I go over and we start talking, and the name "Tim Richmond" comes up. He was a famous race car driver who died of AIDS. *Days of Thunder* with Tom Cruise was made after him.

This guy I was talking to is married for 21 years and has two grown daughters. He goes out and picks up young boys and has sex with them. He couldn't believe that I had AIDS because I look so healthy. He chooses the boys that look healthy. Now he's worried that he might have infected his wife.

When I get dressed up in heels, mini skirt, and makeup, I get hit on all the time. I tell them right out I have AIDS. They say, 'Oh yeah, right.' They think I'm telling them that so they will leave me alone.

This one guy I was dating never used condoms before. All of a sudden he has to use a condom with me. It did not work for him. We tried the female condom. I hated it, he hated it. It's hard to use and it makes a lot of noise. It's like fucking a hefty bag. We couldn't have sex because he would lose his erection. But that wasn't the only reason the relationship ended. I've had my hysterectomy so I'm not going to have PMS ever again. (PMS—Putting up with Men's Shit.)

Mortality-wise, I think I'm too mean to die.

monica johnsen

31, HIV positive since 1984, diagnosed in 1989, infected through a blood transfusion

I received a letter from the blood bank saying that the transfusion I was given a few years earlier contained blood from an HIV positive donor who had died from AIDS. I went and was tested. The test came back inconclusive—I took this as a "no." Five years later, I'm six weeks pregnant and I go see my Ob-gyn. I tell her about the transfusion and the test I took. She re-tested me and it was positive.

When she actually told me I was positive, I had to decide whether to have the baby or an abortion. I had the baby.

My doctor was really supportive. She didn't know a lot about HIV and pregnancy, but she found out as much as she could. She is the same doctor I have today. I had my baby—I had a C-section because he had not turned.

His name was Vaurice LaMon. When he was five or six months old he had thrush. We went to C100 in New Orleans. They have a leper colony there and they were able to do some cultures. It was right before Christmas. The doctors there said he would develop AIDS and not live to be one.

After I cried for several days I went to see my pediatrician. My son was the only HIV patient she had. She said she was not God; she was only a doctor. She said I had to pray. So we prayed together.

After the thrush, he did well for awhile. On his one-year birthday we went back to show the doctor he made it.

Shortly after that visit he got pneumonia and lost all his motor skills. Then he progressed quickly. He lived till he was three and a half. He was sick a lot. We had birthday parties every month. We had 25 years worth of birthday parties in his three years. We took pictures at home every day.

Dr. Dyess, our pediatrician, was really supportive. I dreaded the hospital stays. She would let us drive back and forth so he didn't have to stay overnight. She worked on

82

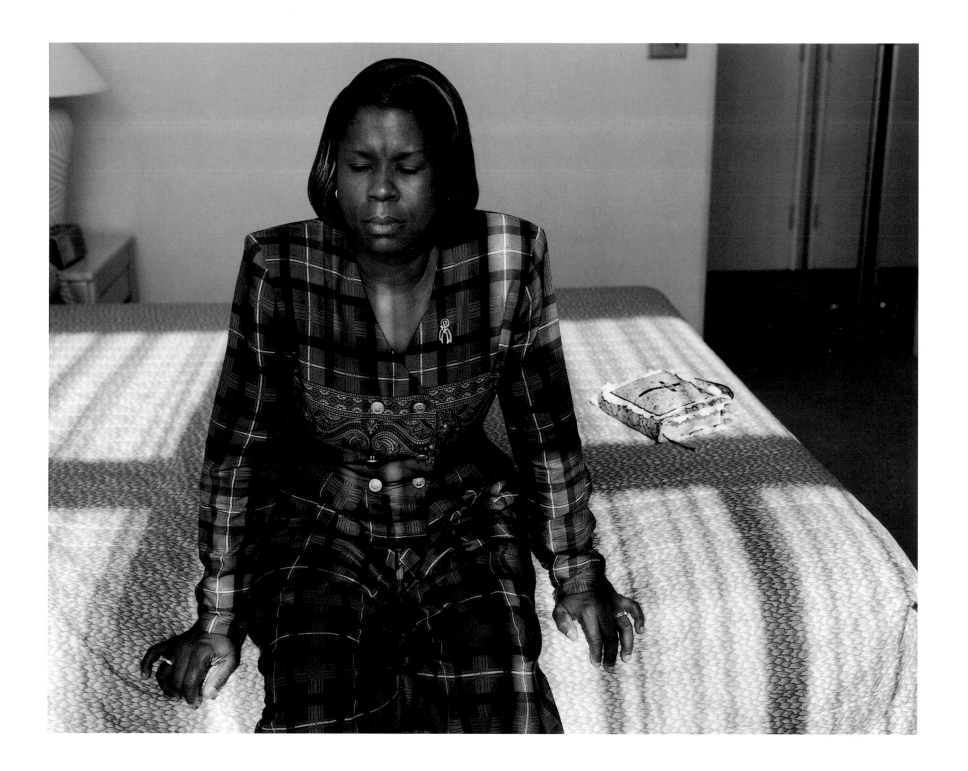

several occasions to help us stay out of the hospital. Sometimes he would just have to stay.

I can't say enough about Dr. Dyess.

When Vaurice was two she arranged a trip to Disney World for me and my son. We stayed for a week. For his third birthday he had a private party at the Barney studio because he was a big Barney fan. We are still good friends. If I'm having problems with my doctor I talk to her about it.

Vaurice died September 28, 1993. It was a Tuesday. He went into the hospital on Sunday. They put him in ICU. He was having congestive heart failure. He stayed in ICU until Tuesday. They didn't think it was clearing—there was nothing else they could do. They put him on the pediatric floor. He died 2 hours later. He died smiling. I tell people he had a very high pain tolerance. He always smiled, even when he was really hurting.

The nurses and everybody there were so supportive. When he died, Dr. Dyess's office closed for the services because everyone who worked there came. We had a small graveside service. Two hundred people came. It was a very mixed group. You can usually tell a black funeral from a white funeral; with my baby you wouldn't have known which it was.

I was in school that semester. I graduated that December.

After that I was home alone for three months. I was filled with grief.

My younger sister said she would be a surrogate mother so I could have a child. I wouldn't try and have another baby. She got pregnant. It was an unplanned pregnancy. She said that I could adopt this baby. We found out it was a boy. I wanted his name to include Vaurice's middle name, LaMon. I named him Avery before he was born. I wanted something that would match LaMon and that he could spell before he was five.

December 4th Avery was born. I went down to be with my sister while she delivered. My sister was in labor for a long time. She was having problems. Toxemia, I think. Avery ended up having to stay in the hospital for two weeks. He needed to be on an IV. At first it scared me but all my friends who worked in the hospital told me he would be okay.

He was discharged December 18. The day he was discharged was my graduation day. I missed my surprise graduation party because I left to go pick him up as soon as I had that diploma in my hands. I was really excited. When I got there he had already been discharged. I picked him up from my little sister's. We went to Wal-Mart to pick up a few things before I left to go home. I held him that night and cried.

Dr. Dyess knew I had no medical coverage. She made it

clear that she would take care of Avery for free. She and a friend gave me a surprise baby shower before he was even out of the hospital. I got all the big stuff—high-chair, stroller, car seat. Of course the car seat was from Dr. Dyess. That was one of her pet peeves.

It has been wonderful being with Avery. He just turned three. We talk about Vaurice LaMon, his cousin. We pray and tell him, 'Hey.'

He knows my sister gave birth to him. He calls me "mama" and calls her "Titi." He has three siblings, my sister's children. He knows his sisters. He knows my sister had him for me because I couldn't have a baby. Sometimes he calls her mama when he is begging. They know how to work you.

I'm doing good. I've had some problems with the only infectious disease doctor around and finally had to stop seeing him. Saying that Louisiana is only a few years behind in HIV treatment is a mild understatement.

I have a family practitioner that I see. I'm his only HIV patient. We do it together. If I ask him something and he doesn't know the answer, he will find out. I can talk to him. He was the one who told me there is a new infectious disease specialist in town and he wouldn't mind if I wanted to go see him. Initially, I said 'No, I don't feel like trying to break someone else in.' I eventually went, but it didn't last.

He is an infectious disease doctor, not an HIV specialist—he deals with all infectious diseases. We didn't get along very well. He just doesn't get it. When I went to the National Skills Building conference, I attended everything on HIV treatments. I wanted to get educated because of the new viral load testing. I brought back all this literature. He didn't even want to look at it. I wasn't to question anything he said. I was to just do what he told me to do.

I had to go back to Dr. Dyess and ask her if I was being unreasonable. Did I need to stay with him? She knows me and she tells me what I need to hear. I went back to my family practitioner.

I was taking AZT and 3TC but stopped because I didn't see any changes in my blood work. I wanted to do the Chinese medicine but there's nothing like that here.

Actually I'm contemplating having another baby. I had ruled it out when my son was sick but now the statistics are so much better. Before one out of every three babies born to an HIV positve mother would remain HIV positive. Now they have all kinds of treatment and can lower the chances of having a baby that remains infected to seven percent. I know what people might think, it's a personal choice. People have to be there to understand.

I don't think HIV will kill me. I will live however long God intends for me to be here.

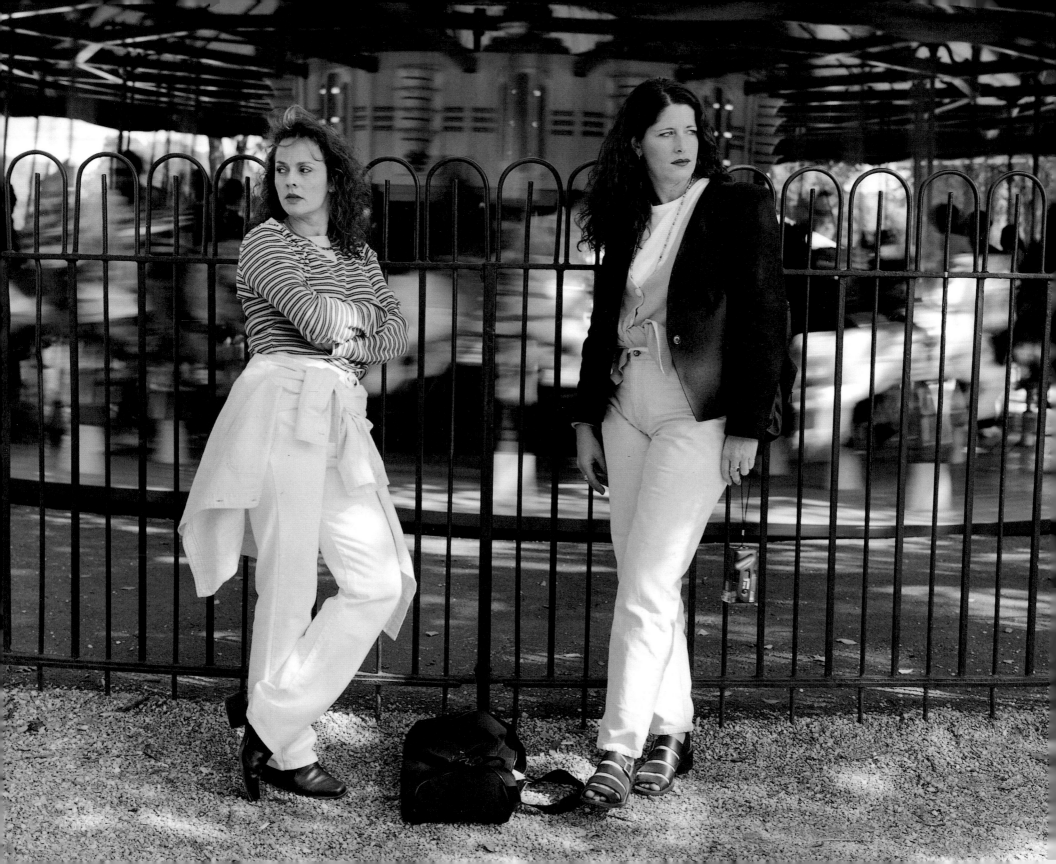

ada arias

36, diagnosed HIV-positive in 1993, infected through sex

sheri kaplin

32, HIV-positive since 1988, diagnosed in 1994, infected through sex

ada: A friend of mine had an experience with a condom breaking and decided that she better get tested for HIV. She went through a week of hell while she waited for the test results. She kept saying she would rather kill herself than have AIDS. This made me start thinking about my own experiences. I had been divorced for the last few years and had unprotected sex. I thought, 'Let me get tested.'

I went to the clinic and they took blood. I was just going through the motions. I was certain I was negative. I wasn't promiscuous. I was young. When I dated, I didn't sleep with anyone till I thought I knew them. I didn't do IV drugs.

I went alone to get the results. They told me that the results came back positive. My first reaction was it was a mistake. They told me they had done an ELISA test and would confirm it with the Western Blot test. The second time I came back to get the results I can't say I was hopeful. I had been thinking, 'Yes, it could be possible.'

The test came back positive. My first question was,

Ada (left) and Sheri each created a support group to address specific needs of women living with HIV.

Before I went public I talked to my family.

They are very educated now about HIV. They talk to me

about medications. If they see a program

on TV they call me and tell me to put the channel on.

They ask questions all the time.

'Where do I go from here? What doctors are informed?' I immediately took action. I wrote to the Center for Disease Control. I didn't want anyone in my family to know that I was getting this information so I put it under my son's name because at the time he wasn't living at home and no one would open his mail. I had told the CDC that he was working on a report on HIV/ AIDS.

I started looking for support. I found a group. I went to two sessions, and there were only three people and the therapist. I was looking for women I could relate to—working women from the Hispanic culture. I told the therapist, 'If you want, I could pull something together. I will make flyers and hand them out in the street.' She brought some of her private clients into the group. I also brought some people. It started to grow. I sent flyers to offices that dealt with HIV-positive women. Some women

came in because of word of mouth. We got to the point where we were 20 to 25 women. We had all types, but we were from the same socio-economic background.

The problem was by the time an hour was up we had just gotten around the circle. A lot of us were not getting what we needed. It was more of a crisis-intervention group. We wanted to go into something deeper. The therapist wanted to keep it as a crisis-intervention session. She was not flexible. That's when Positive Hispanic Women's group was born.

There were about ten Hispanic women in the group. We had already started to meet for dinner. We discussed starting the group. Initially it was a very private group. New members were voted on. It was not publicized.

When I went to the 11th International Conference on HIV/AIDS in Vancouver I became more aware of the needs of Hispanic women. When I returned to the group I said we have to open it up. It's hard for Hispanics to come out because of their culture. Talking in mixed groups of men and women, or with people of another culture, can be difficult. What happens is we don't share deep things. No one was meeting this need in the Miami area. I think it will be going uphill from now on with the organization growing every day.

I just did a fund-raiser and I got sick. It took a toll on me. I had the flu and herpes. I was in the dumps. I decided to take a step back and look objectively at my life. The organization has taught me that I have family and friends who will support me—but if Ada doesn't take care of herself, no one will. I'm striving for balance. Trying to have a good relationship and grow spiritually is hard, but I'm getting there.

I have two boys, 16 and 17. They know I'm

HIV. They don't talk about it. I bring it up whenever I can. I want to reinforce the risks that are out there for them. My family is okay with my diagnosis. Before I went public I talked to my family. They are very educated now about HIV. They talk to me about medications. If they see a program on TV they call me and tell me to put the channel on. They ask questions all the time.

It's important to have the support of family. I remember when I used to keep it under lock and key. Just to read the information was stressful. Before I told anyone, I did all my reading in hiding. I waited till they went to sleep to read it in secret. I sacrificed my own sleep. I made sure not to leave anything out—lock it in the filing cabinet, not leave the key around. I was always sure to get the mail first. I took all my medicines in private. My kids would ask, 'Why are you taking all those vitamins?' Why was I spending so much money on all that stuff? Once, my son saw me spend $80 on Co Q10. He said, 'You could buy me a pair of pants with all that money.' When I went to acupuncture, I lied. How many friends can I see every Wednesday at the same time? So much deception. It was painful.

I came out slowly. I told my boyfriend after three months so he could be tested. In the meantime I kept my distance from him sexually. He was not a live-in boyfriend. I thought for sure that I gave it to him or he gave it to me. He tested negative. It took me nine months to tell my mother. My mother kept it secret for a year. I told my older son, Michael, his brother, Jorge, and their dad after the first year. By the second year the immediate family knew. I felt more empowered. The rest of my family found out when I decided to make the organization public. When we gave this last fund-raiser, two whole tables were filled with family members.

sheri: I founded an agency called Positive Connections. I initially got into it as a way to fulfill my own needs as a straight woman in a gay man's epidemic. I assumed there were others out there like me that needed emotional and social support, as well as a place to learn about all the aspects of AIDS. There is more to staying alive than just popping a pill and getting through this.

Due to my work I'm reminded about HIV every day. It's not because I'm taking pills, physically I feel fine. It's the daily contact with people living with HIV. I see the different stages of the illness up close. It keeps me very grateful for my own health. I was calling to remind people about our Christmas party today. I must have called a hundred people. At least forty or more are sick now. They are at home feeling miserable and there's nothing I can do. They are too young to be so sick.

I have great need to love and nurture. Lately, though, I have not been nursing myself. I have been allowing myself to be consumed. This organization is a business. I had no idea what I was getting myself into when I started this. There are so many people infected and in need of services. AIDS has become an industry.

Before I found out, I never thought of HIV at all. I was with a man for about ten months. We had unprotected sex a handful of times. We usually used a condom. I wasn't worried about AIDS; I was more worried about getting pregnant. He didn't want to use condoms anymore, so I went to the clinic and got birth control pills. While I was there I thought I might as well take an HIV test. Two weeks later my life changed forever.

When they told me the test came back positive, I immediately went into denial. I accused the clinic of mixing my blood with a gay man's. I wasn't a drug user or Haitian. I wasn't gay. I couldn't believe it, no way; I'm only twenty-nine, I want babies and a husband. I felt so dirty, so contagious. I couldn't help wondering how many years I had left.

I went and got a six-pack. I don't even remember driving home. I called my sister—I told her I was dying. She came right over. We sat in denial all night. We were hanging on

*I do want to get married,
to still have that wedding someday. I have
never given up hope. I have been
frustrated because of my limitations.*

the fact that they made a mistake and all I had to do was get re-tested. My boyfriend was supportive in the beginning. He went and was tested. It came back negative. My test remained positive.

I had to learn everything I could about HIV. I needed to control it. I couldn't teach him because I had to teach myself. I tried but it didn't work. He only stayed with me because his mother told him to stay. She said that I needed him. He would steam out the shower after I had been in it. I had my own glass. I felt so fragile and isolated. He never touched me again—forget about safe sex. I decided I'd rather be alone than be treated like this. It was no support; it was abuse. I said good-bye and good luck.

I do want to get married, to still have that wedding someday. I have never given up hope. I have been frustrated because of my limitations. Just today someone took me to lunch. I felt like there was good chemistry, and he is also positive. A case worker at another agency had called me and said, 'I have someone that I'm sending to you. He is cute, you would make a good couple.' I said, 'No way.' Someone is hooking me up for once. That's all I do—match people up. Everyone should be in love. No one should be alone.

I still want a baby. I would have a baby with a healthy man. Not a man with full-blown AIDS. There is enough information out there to prevent transmission to a child. I wouldn't want to subject my baby or myself to death. I wouldn't be that selfish.

I tested positive in 1991. When I worked the streets, I always used a condom. I wouldn't go out on a date if people wouldn't use it. It wasn't about HIV as much as syphilis and gonorrhea.

When I used to get ready to go out, I would smoke angel dust. I would look in the mirror and say, 'If you're HIV, you can take care, you can live a long time.' When I went to get the results, they asked, 'How you gonna take it if you're positive?' But I knew I got it already, just from intuition. When she told me, I just wanted to take care of myself better. It didn't really bother me then and don't bother me now.

I take medication every day. I don't think about it. Thinking too hard will kill you faster. All I do is thank God for another day of living.

I have been really healthy. I haven't worked the streets for four to five years. I haven't done drugs for two years because I want to live. My lover has custody of his two kids. Jessica is four and Joselyn is three. They call me mommy. I stopped because of these children. I want to be able to take care of them. My lover is positive. We both just happen to be HIV-positive. If he was and I wasn't, I would still be with him.

My whole family knows. The first thing I did was tell my mother and sister. They looked at me and said, 'Please take care of yourself and stay off drugs.'

I go every three weeks to see the doctor. I have a great doctor. I'm fine with the medication.

My wish is to have our own house. I would like to finish school to be a nurse. I always wanted to be a nurse. The last grade I went to was the eighth grade. I want to get my GED and work from there.

I'm a really lucky person. I have a good man. I live so much better now than I did before.

sugar

34, diagnosed HIV-positive in 1991, infected through IV drug use

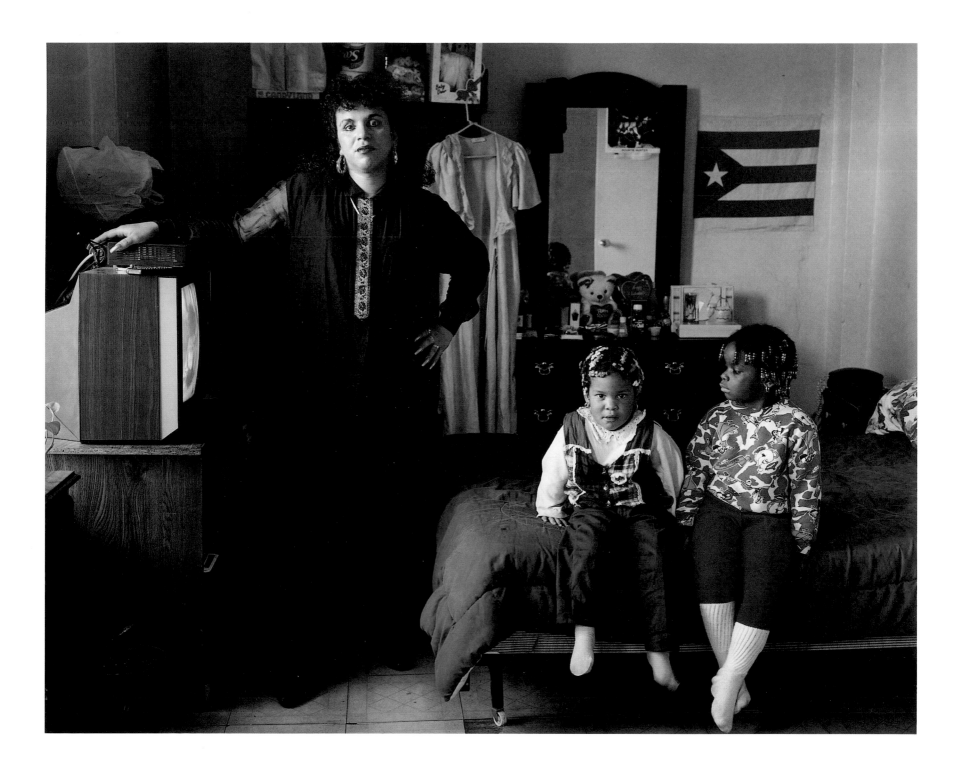

julie evenson

34, HIV-positive since 1989 or earlier, diagnosed in January 1994, infected through sex

I ran into an old boyfriend's grandmother at the grocery store. She was in front of me at the check-out line. It was Christmas-time. We went to the store to get molasses to make ginger-bread cookies. She told me that her grandson was home living with her now. Then she asked if I had heard that he was really sick—he had AIDS. I said, 'No,' and added that it's too bad and that was about it. I was completely stunned, but I don't think it showed. My dad was with me. He heard the whole thing but he didn't say anything. When I got home, I told my mom. She had been watching the kids. She couldn't believe it. I said, 'Do you know what this could mean?' No one believed that I was really at risk. But we were all instantly in another frame of mind. I was scared to death.

The next day I called and made an appointment to take a test. I was so worried and nervous. A week later I went for my results. They called me in and told me I was HIV-positive. I was all alone. The woman was nice but also very nervous. She asked me if I was okay. She said she had never given anyone a positive test result before. I acted as if I was okay. They gave me a lot of information. I just didn't want to believe that it was happening.

I called Troy, my husband, from a pay phone. He could not believe it. He kept saying, 'No way.' I went home and I told my mom. I didn't know what to do. We had to find a place for Troy to go and be tested because the place that I had taken my test was just for women. It's hard for me to remember all this because I blocked a lot of it out. I didn't know anything about AIDS. Magic Johnson had it and that was it. That was all I knew.

Troy was tested and he came back negative. The place that he went to said maybe my test was wrong. They re-tested

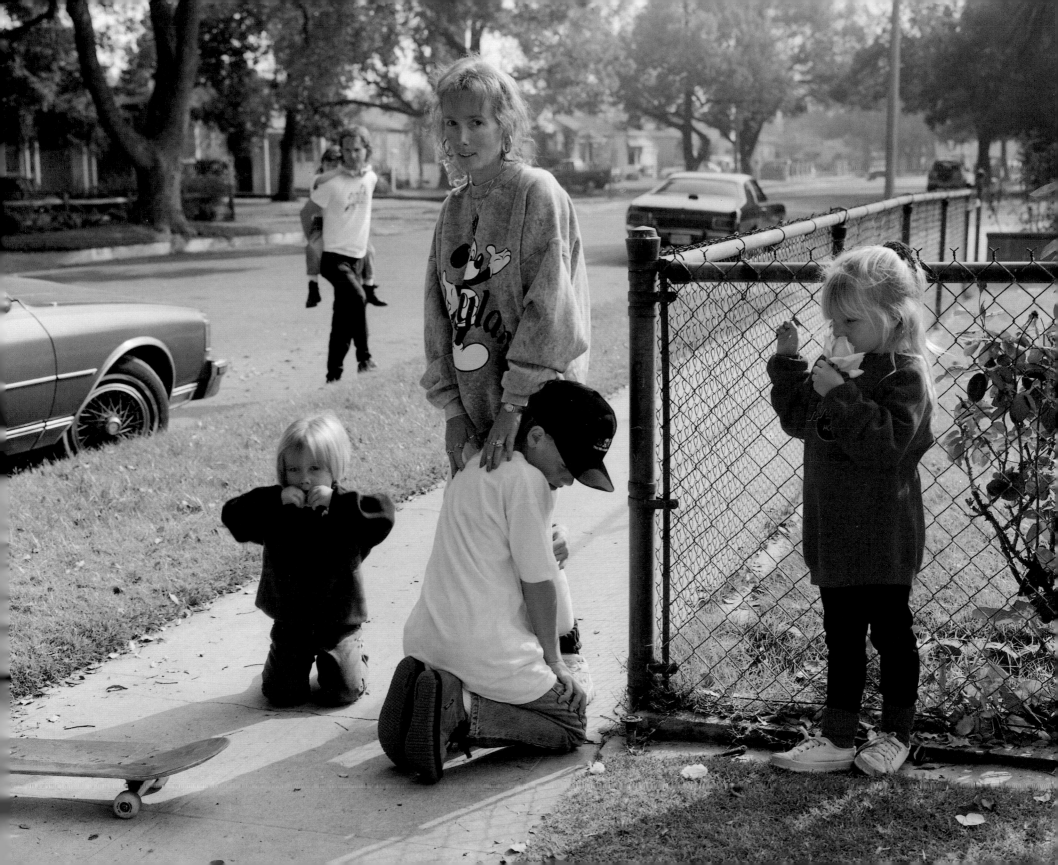

and it was still positive. That was real hard for Troy. When they had said that my test might be wrong, he really got his hopes up. When it still came back positive, he was destroyed. They explained that a man rarely catches it from a woman.

I had to go to some godforsaken clinic somewhere in Hollywood. They were really cold and rude. I wasn't sick and they wanted me to take AZT. I was very anti-drugs. I didn't even take Tylenol. This nurse I saw was just plain mean about it. The only good thing was that she told me I could get all the kids tested at County Hospital.

It was the hardest day in my life. Everyone was nice there. They work a lot with children who are infected. We had the three youngest ones tested. We had to wait three days to find the results. I did a lot of praying and begging. When we returned, it seemed like we waited four or five hours but it was probably only two. I finally went to the desk and asked them why it was taking so long just to get the results to our tests. They said, 'Oh, you're here for the results.' As if they had no idea what was going on. They took me to a waiting room and gave me the results on Christian—he was negative. Chronologically, Madison came next but they skipped her and gave me the results to Myles's test, which was negative. I was in a state of panic because I was certain they were going to say that she was positive. My heart skipped when they said she was negative. They said Myles had to be re-tested because he was only two.

I have had little contact with other people living with AIDS. I met a few people but still continue to do it on my own. I'm not used to asking for any help.

I don't want to take any time from my kids. Every minute I can spend with them counts. Even going to the grocery store. They can sleep with me every night if they want to. That's the best therapy for me.

It took me thirty years to get exactly what I wanted: a great husband, four beautiful children, a house, and a good job. I had it all for about a year and a half, and then I found out and my life fell apart. I'm still happy. I just had to adjust my priorities. I used to be so exact and picky. Everything had to be in place. Now it's more important to be with the kids. To be with people I love.

I didn't tell anyone for a long time. Now I don't care. I told my church, friends, and family. I have gotten positive encouragement even from people I don't know. I haven't told everyone at school because I didn't want my children to suffer. You know how it is: kids can be really cruel and I didn't want mine to be ridiculed. It's hard enough for them as it is. I can't do all the things I would love to do, like play catch or jump on the trampoline. They all know I'm sick but only Ajay really knows what it is.

We were watching a TV special with Magic Johnson. He was talking with kids about AIDS. Ajay asked me, 'Mom, is what you have like AIDS?' I told him that's exactly what it is. I said, 'You can tell anyone you want, but be careful.' I explained to him as best I could all the implications of telling people that his mom has AIDS. He hasn't really told anyone yet.

I tell Ajay everything, and Christian too if he asks. I figure if they can ask the questions, they need to know the answers. My mother gets a little embarrassed when I explain things, especially about sex. She'll say, 'Oh he doesn't need to know that.' Christian hasn't said too much. He is only seven. He didn't know exactly what I had. Well, at least he didn't until you came to visit. When you came and took the pictures, he figured out it was AIDS. After you left, he asked me if I gave it to daddy then would I still have it?

We keep praying for that miracle cure. Myles and Madison know I have a blood disease and that I'm weak and need lots of sleep—which they don't let me get. They don't know what it's called. It hurts sometimes. I will be feeling really awful and Madison will want to play. The other night I told her, 'Mommy doesn't feel well.' She got kind of mad and said, 'Mommy never feels well.'

My mom doesn't tell people. She will say I'm anemic. When I was diagnosed with cancer, she used that for a while. I asked her once, 'Mom are you embarrassed?' She said her friends just wouldn't understand.

After I got out of the hospital with pneumonia, my husband's parents said, 'Oh you're looking much better, you will be good as new in no time.' I said, 'I will never be good as new.' After I told them what was really going on, things changed.

His father used to kiss me on the lips, and now he just hugs me. I'm kind of glad that he just hugs me. I used to hate his kisses. He would hold my face and give me a big old smooch. It was gross. Whenever we go over to their house, his mom serves me separately. Like if there is salsa and dip, she gives me my own little bowl of salsa. My kids eat out of it—they just think that she gave it to me so it would be easier for me to reach. I know what is really going on and I don't care. That's their problem. They just say, 'Hang in there,' or something like that. If they ask how I'm doing, I don't tell them. I just say, 'Fine.' I never get into how I really feel. That would be pretty funny: 'Well I can barely see anymore, I puke up almost everything that I try to eat, it's excruciating to walk because all my limbs are completely numb, and I feel like I'm about to pass out I'm so tired. Other than that, I'm fine. How are you?' The bottom line is you never feel good. Some days are good days compared to the bad days but those good days are few and far between.

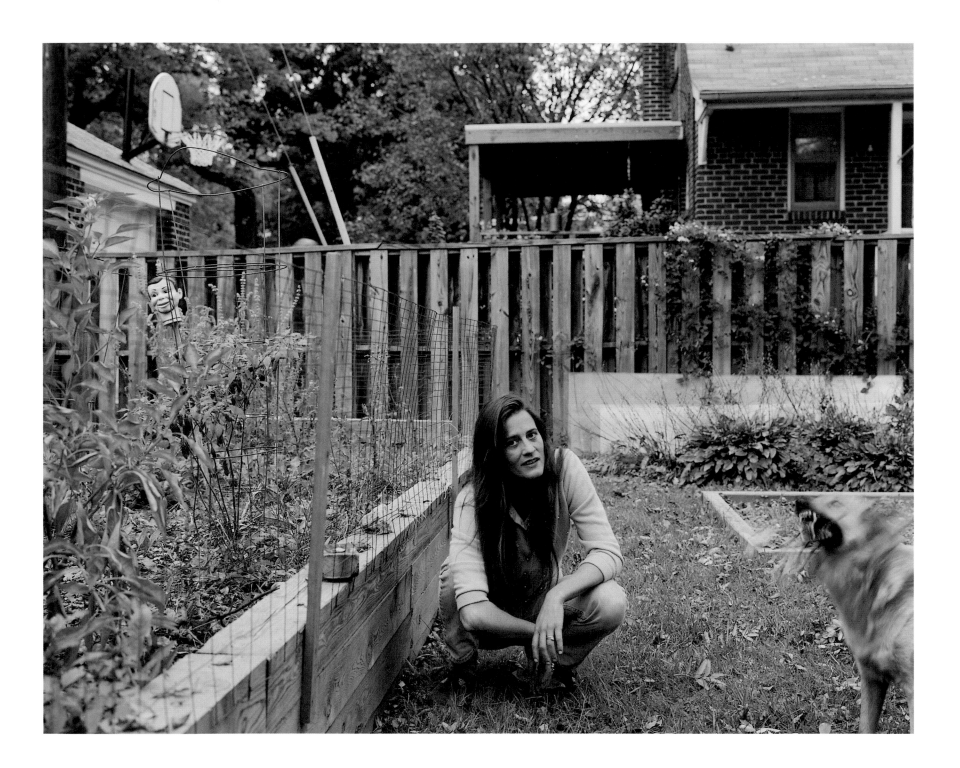

I'm sick and tired of saying I feel sick. I'm on Saquinavir, Ritonavir, 3TC, and d4T. I was in a clinical trial that was supposed to be this regimen. After they unblinded the study I found out that I was only taking d4t. I was angry. I went on the Crixivan and the 3TC but I couldn't comply. I just couldn't do it. I ended up stopping, then I couldn't go back on because of resistance. Doing the regimen I'm on now was not an overnight decision. I had to ask myself, 'Can I do this; be committed?' I prayed for the willingness. In the meantime I ended up with shingles and respiratory problems. I kept getting all these infections, even though my counts weren't that bad. I went back and forth. It took a year and a half of strange bacterial infections before I decided to do it. I'd been waiting till my viral load reached a certain point, but it was getting ridiculous. I was having symptoms of AIDS. It has been a major decision for

both my husband and I. We are banking on all the hype— that it will give you a beautiful life. Truth is, I don't feel real beautiful puking my guts up and having diarrhea. I couldn't even let Steve, my husband, touch me. I'm feeling so yucky.

I'm blessed with a good doctor, Dr. Gallant. He is well informed about AIDS. He's been working in the field since the eighties. He's someone who is willing to talk to me. I have other issues besides HIV but they affect HIV.

One of them is bulimia. With this new regime I have to eat a lot of fat. It's a scary thought. I need to change everything from zero fat to total fat. I eat eggs and bacon now. Before it was like, 'Fat! Oh my God!' I don't even have fat in my pancake mix. You need fat to absorb the drug. The good thing is these drugs are less regimented. I only have to take them at nine in the morning and nine at night. I have such an aversion to food when I take my meds. When I had

laurie priddy

32, diagnosed HIV-positive in 1990, infected through sex

to take them in the middle of the day it was excruciating. I never ate. You must eat to take the drug. I've had to learn to love food.

Dr. Gallant treats the entire person not just the virus. They are not separate. He asks about what is going on in my whole life, then he asks how I am feeling physically and what is happening to me regarding HIV. That way he can see when it's stress affecting my health or HIV.

I don't sit on the exam table till it's time. I sit in the chair. Being on the table you feel like the sick patient. Your feet are dangling, you're vulnerable. He could push a button and I could go flying.

Having AIDS is a head thing.

When I say I'm not feeling good someone always seems to say, 'But you look great, you look wonderful.' Sometimes I feel like I shouldn't tell them how I really feel. It seems like they don't want to believe me since I look all right. These days, I say I feel so awful so much that I'm afraid people will say, 'Oh God, she's sick again.'

Last week I went out on the motorcycle. I feel afraid that people will judge me. If I'm that sick I shouldn't be doing that. It's the one thing that makes me feel normal. It's the physicalness of getting on the motorcycle. I put my leather

on and I feel strong. I braid my hair back and I look cool.

I don't want to live my life lying in bed all the time. Even Steve doesn't argue anymore. He doesn't get alarmed. He allows me to be sick and do what I think is necessary for my well-being. He would coddle me but he knows that's not what I need.

First time I ever saw him, I told my friend, 'That's my type of guy.' I was attracted to his whole person—a combination of soft and manly.

Shortly after I met him, I went to bike week in Daytona. I was invited to stay at a house where Steve was staying. I knew he was there, but it didn't mean anything because I also knew he had a girlfriend.

I got there and I was the only woman in the house. The four other guys watched over me. They were my personal bodyguards, making sure I didn't get a tattoo on my forehead or something. Instead, I got one on my ankle, and they all got one too. I remember that night. We were at this big biker bar and I'm in this trailer with this guy who is ten sheets to the wind. The guys were all singing 'It's the midnight special.' I felt pretty, feminine, and desirable, and HIV wasn't with us. It was great. Steve kept trying to get me to ride with him but I was too giddy. A part of me wanted to be wrapped around him and another part was scared. Like in high school: you want to know if he likes you, but then he might not; so you don't want to know. I also knew he had a girl and I didn't want to get involved with that. Later, I found that he was attracted to me and he was getting ready to end his relationship. He hadn't been happy and wanted to move on.

I went to give a lecture on HIV in Seattle. When I returned to Baltimore, I got off the plane, and Steve was waiting for me in the airport. I had been flying for eight hours. I was a mess. I definitely had picked up the grunge look. He was so sexy, I couldn't imagine him standing there for me. He said, 'I've come to take you to dinner.' He took me down to Annapolis and we had dinner. I had a little hesitation. I told him that my car's here. He said, 'Just leave it. Your friends will bring you here tomorrow to pick it up.' I was red in the face, sweating. My underwear was sticking. I felt like I had to go to the ladies room and find one of those blowers.

He knew I was HIV from friends. I didn't have to introduce it into the relationship. It shouldn't make a difference, but it does. I didn't have to go through "I have something to tell you." I might be completely secure with it but when I have to tell someone, this blow-up vest inflates around me.

It keeps me secure. I get cocky, like, 'I have this, I handle it, so get over it.' Inside, you're scared. You can call them an ignorant motherfucker if they say the wrong thing but the hurt doesn't go away.

It happened so quick for us. I felt like, 'I found you!' He felt the same way. He ended up asking me to marry him after dinner one night. I remember feeling like all my predictions about the future had been wrong. I couldn't believe this was really, truly happening. I just sat there. I didn't say 'Yes' right away. Later, he told me he felt like he was going to have to go looking for rope to hang himself. I was playing with my food. I would say, 'Really?' There was a little part of me that felt like I didn't deserve all this good stuff. I told him, 'Yes.'

We spotted each other in August, met in April, he proposed in July, and we married in September. When people ask him about us he says, 'Your forever is not the same as our forever.'

I want it to be way longer. I have told him that. He said once, 'I never wanted to have children but for the first time I've met someone who I want to be the mother of my child.' That is saying so much more to me than 'You're beautiful and sexy.' I do this medicine for Steve. I don't mean it as a burden with all the side effects. I just want to be with him for a long time.

tammy brisco

26, diagnosed HIV-positive in 1994, infected through sex

I went in for a routine exam. I had just been divorced. The doctor asked me if I was dating. I said, 'Yes.' He asked if I wanted to be tested for a series of things, HIV being one of them. The first test came back abnormal. I was in my window period. It didn't show an absolute positive, just a possibility. I went to the health department. They gave me another test. This one came back definitely positive.

The doctor walked into the room and announced, 'You're HIV-positive, any questions? No? Okay.' That was it. Total numbness—that's the best I can describe it. I had so many reactions I had none. He just walked out of the room and left me sitting there.

I paid my bill and left. As I was driving back to work, I broke down.

At one point I went to get my boyfriend. I needed moral support. I was dazed and crying. I was working, and still am, as an administrative assistant in Chaves County. I told my co-workers I wouldn't be in for the rest of the day. A couple of my co-workers knew I was getting tested. They didn't ask any questions. Whatever it was they could tell by just looking at me and it warranted me being gone.

We drove to a park and talked. He tried to comfort me. He told me that it wasn't the end of the world. At the time it seemed like it was.

It was in the back of both of our minds that he might be positive but neither one of us wanted to address it. He refused to be tested for a few weeks. His attitude was, 'There is nothing I can do, why find out to just worry.'

I finally convinced him that it was important. His test came back positive. He came immediately to my office and told me. He was very upset.

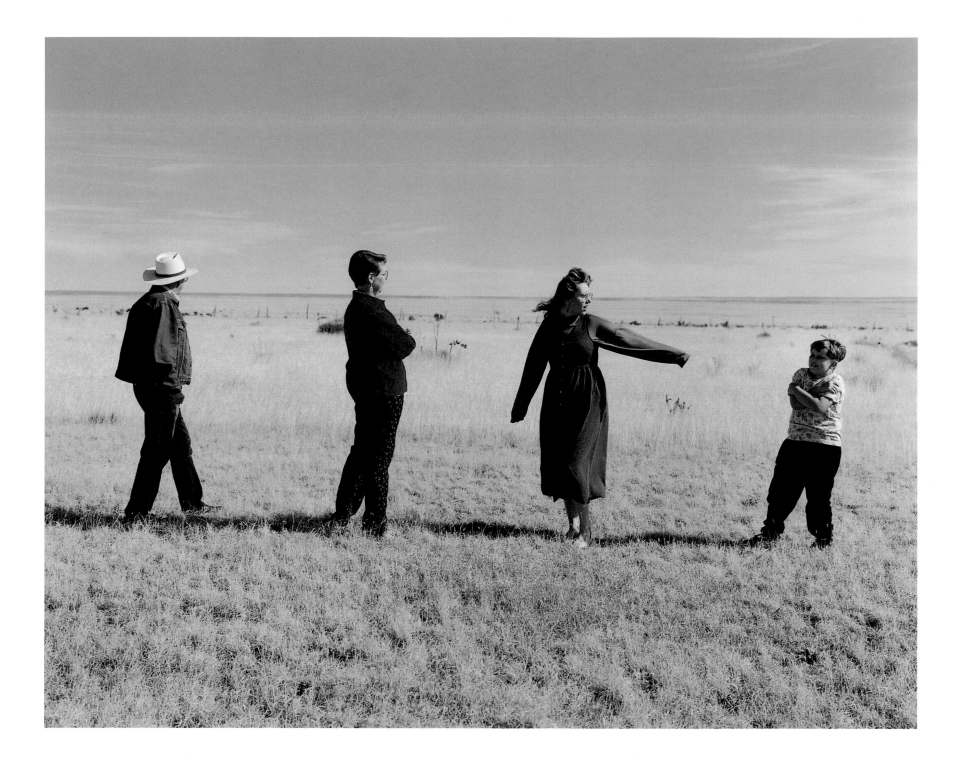

We never really pointed blame on one or the other. It didn't do any good. It was something we were going to handle together.

Then I had to tell my family. It was around Christmas. I didn't want to tell them because of the holidays. But that only lasted about two or three days. It was killing me holding in this enormous secret. I told my mom. She knew that something was wrong anyway. She kept saying, 'Are you all right? Please tell me what's wrong.' We're really close. While we were alone I told her. She hadn't even known I was taking the test, so it was a real shock to her. She started crying. We held each other a long time. Then she asked me if I knew who gave it to me. At that point I didn't.

She asked if I told anyone else, and I said 'No.' She just talked about my feelings, how I was doing, what my plans were, did I have to take any drugs, who was my doctor. That sort of thing.

She asked if I wanted to tell the rest of the family together. We decided to wait. We didn't want to ruin Christmas.

After I came home I told her it was okay if she wanted to tell the family. She shared it with more family than I anticipated. I thought, 'immediate family.' I didn't realize she would tell second cousins, distant family. The notifying came in phases. Different people learned at different times. I got cards from family I met only once or twice. It was helpful, since I didn't have immediate family in the town where I lived.

My dad didn't want to discuss it. If it was brought up he got very angry. My dad is a very unemotional man. That, and the fact that he can do nothing to help me get over this, makes him very angry. To some extent he still avoids the subject though he is getting a lot better.

My daughter, Ashley, was seven at the time. She was the first person I told after my boyfriend. Being as young as she was, it was hard for her to comprehend. The only thing I could think of to tell her was, 'If mommy gets hurt and is bleeding, you must stay away from her and just go get help.' She understood that but accepting it was hard. Now she knows more. I answer any question she has. When the subject of sex comes up I explain in simple answers on her level. I tell her I was infected by unprotected sex. It's a lot for her but it's the only way I can explain it. She knows what sex is. I have a book called *How I Was Born*, and it has pictures. She gets scared for me even if I get the slightest cold. I never used to get sick. If I have to stay home from

I have joined the Speaker's Bureau.

I travel all over and speak to people about my experience.

I think people identify with me.

They can see HIV is not just a gay-man or drug-users disease.

work, she is afraid I will not be there when she gets back.

The challenge comes with my four year old, Jaushua. I have to explain why he can't use mommy's toothbrush, 'Mommy is sick.' Trying to explain a sickness that isn't about coughing and taking medicine is hard but at his age he can't understand much more.

I'm still with my boyfriend. He was the first and only man I have been with after I was divorced. I believe now that I was infected by him. He's not sure how he got it. He doesn't like to talk about it. We have protected sex. My mom still lectures me that celibacy is a good thing. I think she wants to encourage me that it's okay to not have sex.

I was married in 1990 and divorced in February of 1995. We were right in the middle of divorce when I found out. My ex-husband was angry and scared. He

asked if he could have it. I said there was that chance.

I see my ex-husband on a weekly basis to exchange our son, Jaushua. He shared that he went and got tested, and it was negative. We are on good terms now. He is supportive. Every once in a while he says he keeps me in his prayers, and he is always quick to share any news he hears about HIV.

I feel different than when I was first diagnosed. I feel in control because if I don't think like that, then the virus will do what it wants. I have joined the Speaker's Bureau. I travel all over and speak to people about my experience. I think people identify with me. They can see HIV is not just a gay-man or drug-users disease.

For the most part I have always been a positive person. When I'm not speaking or at a meeting regarding HIV, I just live as I did before but with more focus with the important things in life, like my kids.

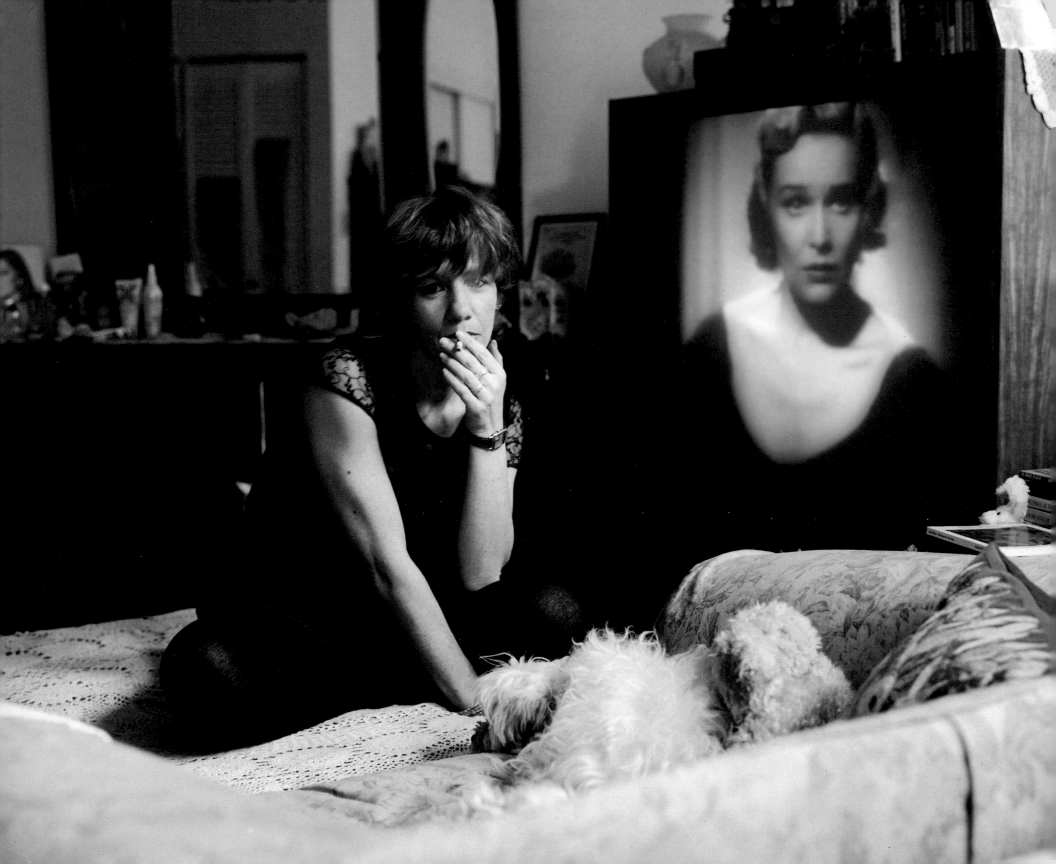

There is no shame, or there should be no shame, in how you get AIDS. AIDS was not sent here to kill us but to waken the humanity in us and help us experience compassion without judgment.

I tested positive on November 6, 1986. I'm assuming I have been positive since 1983. Something was going on. It was like a new phenomenon. I started losing friends to endocarditis. All these people were dying in their early twenties. I had gotten clean in a twelve-step program. My sponsor in the program died of spinal meningitis but people would whisper that it was really AIDS.

I felt plagued by this disease even before I knew for sure that I had it. I would be in the shower and all of a sudden I would be talking to myself and AIDS would come into my mind like some kind of powerful mantra. It was too painful not to know. I suspected I could be positive. Everything that I heard about AIDS I could apply to myself. Still, I was shocked when I actually found out. It's different thinking you might be infected and having someone confirm that reality.

I had not had a drug or a drink for 13 months when I went to get tested. It was some place out in Queens where no one would know me. I made arrangements to go with a guy that I knew had already been diagnosed positive.

I was waiting in this little room with pukey green tiles on the walls. Everybody had their head down No one was looking at anyone. Finally they called out my number. I went into the office. This man looked at me from behind his desk. He said he was sorry. I cut him right off and I said, 'You don't have to say anything.' He said, 'There are some things that you need to know. First of all, this is not a death sentence.' At that point, I turned and looked out the window. My life

robin horowitz

40, HIV-positive since 1983, diagnosed in November 1986, infected through IV drug use

I don't bring a virus to a relationship;

I bring the enlightenment in my life, my passion and lust for living.

I'm not some giant virus walking around on

two legs. Sex and intimacy are more than exchanging fluids.

became calm. Everything disappeared like a 'pre'-anger or something. I was thinking I was angry but I was really scared and alone.

I went right from the testing site to a place where I knew I could get some dope. I went on a run for the next four months. That night I went home with this guy I just met. My boyfriend of six years came over and found us in bed. He could tell I was definitely high. I had left my works out on the table. I was very flippant and just told him, 'By the way, I have AIDS.'

The next day I begged him to take me back but I knew it was over, and it was. His only concern was if he was positive. I had really low self-esteem. I was the bad person. I felt so guilty. It was easier to worry about him. So I joined his turmoil to avoid mine. After that run I began reevaluating, rearranging, and prioritizing my life.

I had a successful corporate career. I had built that career at the expense of pursuing dreams as a ballet dancer and a writer. I decided to give up my house, my Mercedes, and go to Miami. In Miami, I wrote and published a book called *As Flesh Turns to Angels*. It was a series of poems and journal entries about letting go of the physical attachment, letting go of the body, and pursuing a spiritual life. My life up to this point had been one of distraction.

My parents always expected greatness from me but never applauded me when I attained it. I was an athlete, I modeled, I did well in school. My dad valued money, my mom had an IQ of 220. She was brilliant, but could not relate to me as a child. I never felt safe or centered. The society I lived in told me to go after dreams but then they told me what my dreams should be: a new car, a husband, a career with security. It was all about building walls and isolation. The more attachments that I acquired, the more separated from other human beings I became.

We have gone in a direction away from humanity. We forgot the spirit lives forever and we need nourishment for our souls. We talk out of both sides of our mouth. We are told to do the right thing, love your brother, and then we are taught to look out for ourselves and step on who you have to. Don't give away secrets. People live two lives. To me you can't go to your church on Sunday, and Monday to Friday do your own thing. We need to be spirit-directed not ego-directed. The whole motive of ego is to keep us engaged about the next man, next job, next good thing. I never knew a person who finally got to their death bed and said, 'I'm so glad I got that Mercedes. It was a much better choice than that Porsche.' I have always felt like this but I didn't find the urgency to speak before I had HIV.

When my boyfriend left, it was a relief. I didn't want to be with him, but it set off a lot of self-esteem issues. I'm wasn't ready to deal with rejection and I'm not willing to settle for anyone just because I'm HIV-positive. HIV can expand and widen potential intimacy; not make it smaller. I don't bring a virus to a relationship; I bring the enlightenment in my life, my passion and lust for living. I'm not some giant virus walking around on two legs. Sex and intimacy are more than exchanging fluids.

Since I have been diagnosed

I have had some great sex and some lousy attempts at relationships. I don't know if it's just HIV that makes it difficult for me to find a partner. I'm selective and cautious. I want a multi-dimensional person. In *The Prophet*, Kahlil Gibran says, 'Whatever has been carved out has left a space that has deepened you.' I want to meet someone who is deeply carved.

I'm told HIV is not a death sentence. I don't know what they think of death, but death to me is an ending of what I had previously known. HIV put an end to the life that I had previously known. I was infected when I was thirty. That is the beginning of adulthood. It's the beginning of hope for the future and being your own pilot. It's as if 29 years of planning was pulled out from under me. I made a decision to change the way I thought rather than adjust to AIDS. AIDS eradicated my belief system. I had to learn that every ending is a beginning. Death is freedom from the bondage of a physical body.

brenda

35, diagnosed HIV-positive in 1994, infected through sex

My husband, Steve, had been very sick. We didn't know what was wrong. We had been going to different emergency rooms for about six months. I think that he knew but he wouldn't tell me. I thought he had pneumonia. He was coughing all the time and running a fever. He hadn't been taking care of himself and he was still taking drugs. All through this time he had never tried to stop using.

He started doing drugs a few years after we were married. In the beginning it wasn't the primary thing in his life. I didn't know what he was doing. His moods would change. He would take things from the house and always be borrowing money. I thought about him getting HIV and we talked about it. Once he asked me to be tested and I refused because I was afraid to find out the results. I had it in the back of my mind but I really didn't think that I was infected because I was healthy. I had four healthy children, 16, 15,

12, and 7. We were together 18 years and married 9.

He became so ill we had to admit him to Brookdale Hospital. He was there awhile and then they released him to Linroc Nursing Home. I still didn't know how serious it was until then. He lost his ability to walk and was confined to a wheelchair. When I would go to see him he would act like he would be getting out soon. Then he became very disoriented. The doctors told me he had dementia.

I still did not know that he had AIDS. One time I was visiting and a doctor told me that I should be tested. I asked her, 'Why?' She said that they had tested my husband's blood and he had tested positive for HIV, and right now he is in the late stages of AIDS. I don't know if she was supposed to tell me. He still had not told me and by then we couldn't talk about it because he was not able to really speak or understand what was going on because of the dementia.

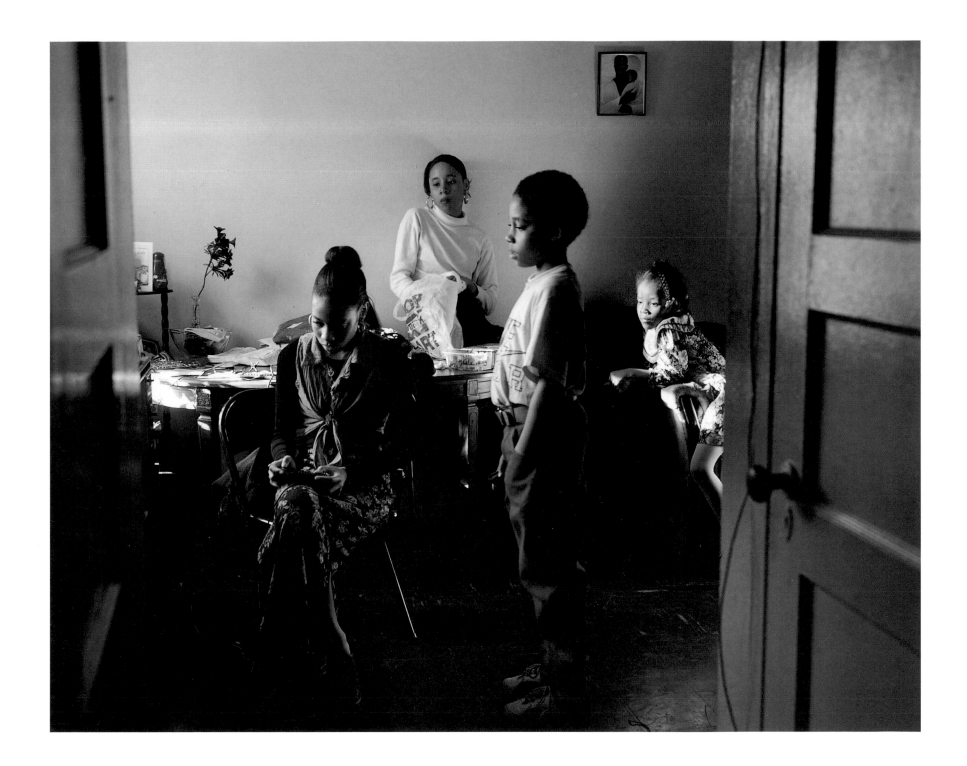

I went to a clinic and was tested. The test came back positive. At first I was shocked. I couldn't accept it and I stayed in denial. I was at a new job and I couldn't explain it to anyone. I had a lot of fear especially as far as my children were concerned.

I was so angry at him. We talked but by then I couldn't get any answers because he was so sick. Still I asked him, 'Why didn't you tell me sooner? Why did you give it to me? Why didn't you protect me?' I don't think he wanted me to get it but he never did anything to stop it. I was so angry—sometimes I didn't want to see him at all.

Still I went to see him as much as I could. I would take the kids but they would get upset. He stayed for a year. I gave him what I could to make him comfortable. Near the end he was admitted twice to Brookdale. The first time I thought he was doing better.

I came in the room and he was sitting up drinking a soda and eating. The second time he went into a coma. He looked so bad. His looks seemed to have deteriorated overnight. His whole body was eaten away. I couldn't look at him. They told me they wanted to do an operation and I said I didn't want them cutting him up. It was obvious that he was not going to make it. I felt like they were just experimenting with him.

I was at work when the doctor called. He said Steve passed away at 12 that day. I was so upset. We made funeral arrangements. My family was there. They helped me through it. It was such a shock to see him dropped into the ground. The kids were very upset.

My son was angry for a long time. He was angry he had left him the way he did They didn't know he was taking drugs. They were upset that he had AIDS, and now they are afraid for me. If I'm sick, they get scared. My oldest daughter stays with me more than she used to. He was a good father. He wasn't a good provider but he stayed with them while I worked. I have forgiven him. It was hard. I stayed angry a long time. At times I felt if he were alive I would kill him for this. I don't deserve it.

...a doctor told me that I should be tested.

I asked her, 'Why?' She said that they had tested my husband's blood

and he had tested positive for HIV,

and right now he is in the late stages of AIDS.

I have educated the children about HIV. They understand it. They want me to stop cigarettes. They know I take medications. We don't talk about it too much. This guy comes to the house and gives them interviews. He asks them all kinds of questions: 'How is your life? How are things affecting you?' The kids get paid fifteen dollars. It also helps them understand HIV better.

Mainly I got information from booklets from the clinics. I went to support groups and I started to adjust. I went to Brookdale and I signed up with their clinic. I had a T-cell count done. It was 250. That was two years ago. They started me with ddI and AZT and some vitamins. It made me feel terrible: insomnia, nausea, and headaches. I felt worse than when I started to take medications. I was very agitated. Now I am taking Zerit, Invirase, and Epivir. I feel much better than being on AZT. I also take golden seal and aloe vera.

Emotionally I'm a lot better. I am going on with my life. I am not in mourning as much. I'm going to church and I'm trying to get on with my life. I hope that they will find a cure. I would like to get a house, move out of these projects, continue working, and someday see my grandchildren born.

glossary

Alcoholics Anonymous (A.A.)—is fellowship of men and women who have the desire to stop drinking. They follow a set of principles laid out in twelve steps.

Acupuncture—is a gentle, non-toxic method of healing that strives to create balance in the body while strengthening all the systems of the body. It is the first most utilized alternative therapy among people with HIV.

AZT—also known as Retrovir (zidovudine) is a anti-viral medication, more specifically, a reverse transcriptase inhibitor. It is thought to be active against HIV by entering infected CD4 cells and keeping the virus from replicating by disturbing the job of an HIV enzyme called reverse transcriptase. There is a lot of controversy about AZT. Burroughs Wellcome Co. (now known as Glaxco-Wellcome) put out the drug in 1987 at the same time they put out the HIV testing kits. They then began a large advertising campaign to get people to go and be tested for the HIV virus. So now if you tested positive, whether you had symptoms or not, there was a drug you could take, AZT. Needless to say, they made millions. The only problem was that there was never any conclusive testing that showed AZT effectiveness in the long run. In recent studies, AZT taken alone has been shown to have only temporary benefit to a small number of people. One of the other problems with AZT is that it has such strong side effects that it could actually mimic some of the symptoms of HIV infection such as nausea, severe headache, and anemia. It has also been linked with lymphoma. AZT at this point has many sister drugs—ddI, ddC, 3TC, and d4T. They work in a similar fashion to AZT. It has become popular to do different combination of these drugs plus protease inhibitor.

Antiviral Medications—is a reference to the drugs listed above.

Bactrim—is a prophylaxis used to prevent PCP pneumonia.

CDC—is the Centers for Disease Control and Prevention. Based in Atlanta, it is a federal government agency that monitors disease in America.

CMV—cytomegalovirus is a common virus related to the herpes simplex virus. CMV usually remains inactive in healthy people. The virus lives in the blood cells and often multiplies when the CD4 count is less than 100. The infection causes fever, fatigue, and weight loss, and resembles mononucleosis. Often symptoms are mild or absent. CMV is a systemic disease which means it can occur throughout the body. In persons with HIV infection, CMV can infect the central nervous system. It can also infect the lungs causing pneumonia. In the brain it can cause swelling of the brain tissue. In the colon it can cause cramps and diarrhea. Hepatitis results from CMV of the liver.

CMV retinitis—inflammation of the retina occurs in as many as a quarter of people with HIV infection and is the most common form of CMV infection. Symptoms include vision changes, floaters, or tunnel vision.

Crixivan—is a brand of protease inhibitor developed by Merck. Also known as indinavir and MK-639.

Chinese medicine—is a system of healing that treats the whole person. This means the physical as well as emotional components. It includes herbs and acupuncture.

Dapsone—is a prophylaxis used to prevent PCP pneumonia.

DES—is a New York State agency that gives financial support to people living with AIDS.

Dementia—happens when HIV infects the brain and other parts of the nervous system. At first, mild abnormalities are detected with careful testing. Later patients may develop difficulty in concentrating, poor memory, slowness in thinking, and inability to perform tasks. Loss of coordination, weakness, and trouble walking may follow. In the most advanced form, a person is bedridden and cannot control bladder or bowels.

Diflucan—is a medication used for candidisis and thrush.

d4T—is a class of anti-retrovirals similar to AZT.

ELISA Test—tests for HIV antibodies. It is a very sensitive test ands is prone to false positives. If you test positive for the ELISA you will generally then be given a Western Blot test which is more specific.

Endocarditis—is a bacterial infection of the heart. Many IV drug users are prone to this infection.

Epstein Barr—is a herpes-like virus that causes mononucleosis—a disorder known for causing extreme fatigue.

MAC—Mycobacterium Avium Complex ordinarily causes local infections of skin and lymph nodes or causes lung infections in persons with preexisting lung disease. HIV infection allows these organisms to spread to other areas of the body.

National Skills Building Conference—is one of the many AIDS conferences that occur on a yearly basis. It helps keep health practitioners as well as people living with AIDS/HIV to stay updated on the most recent developments in the treatment of AIDS as well as how to cope and deal with running AIDS organizations.

Native Medicines—is a system of treatment on the basis of love, hope, faith, and charity. It originated with Native Americans. It includes prayers, ceremonies, and herbs.

Narcotics Anonymous (NA)—follows the same principles as Alcoholics Anonymous but the members may have addictions to drugs as well as alcohol.

Opportunistic illness—opportunistic infections, diseases, and conditions are a group of illnesses that the CDC has used to define AIDS. Many of these diseases have been around for awhile. Some were fairly common such as bacterial pneumonia, and others up until the recognition of HIV infection were relatively rare such as Kaposi's Sarcoma. These illnesses may look like the same diseases as in the past but because they are present in a system that has a weakened immune system they can be life-threatening. In the beginning they looked at what seemed most common among the people who were HIV-positive, who were sick or who had died. They came up with this group of illnesses. There are many other infections that are not on their list, especially when it comes to women and children. Most of their findings were based on men. It took up until 1993 for them to add two diseases that were specific to women—cervical cancer and bacterial pneumonia. They also added recurrent chronic yeast infections as a symptom.

Peripheral neuropathy—this is a general term for any disease of the peripheral nerves—those that control muscles and sensation. Symptoms include burning pain (especially in the feet), loss of sensation, numbness, tingling, and muscle weakness or even paralysis.

PCP—pneumocystis carinii pneumonia is the most common and one of the most deadly infections facing people who are HIV-positive. Pneumocystic carinii is a common microscopic organism that rarely causes disease in people with normal immune systems but can cause havoc in the lungs of people with HIV infection. Early warning signs are fatigue and shortness of breath. As the infection intensifies, rapid breathing, dry-cough, fevers, chills, night sweats, and weight loss can occur.

Protease inhibitors—is a class of drugs developed specifically for the treatment of HIV infection. As this book goes to print, this treatment is classified as experimental, temporary, and expensive to the degree it is exclusive.

PML—progressive multifocal leukoencephalopathy is a brain disorder. Early signs are headache, forgetfulness, double vision, and difficulty walking or speaking. More serious symptoms include loss of vision, seizures, and paralysis.

Prozac—is an anti-depressant drug.

Q10—is a non-prescription compound that claims to help heal the immune system. It can be found in most health-food stores.

Recovery—a term used in Alcoholics Anonymous and other twelve-step programs to indicate a person has stopped using the drug of their choice and is trying to change the lifestyle that so often keeps a person addicted.

Ritonavir—a brand of protease inhibitor developed by Abbot also known as Norvir and ABT-538.

Saquinivir—is a brand of protease inhibitor developed by Hoffman-La Roche. Also known as Invirase and RO-31-8959.

Seroconversion—is the process by which someone goes from being HIV-negative to HIV-positive or HIV-positive to HIV-negative. When a person is exposed to HIV the body creates antibodies to fight the invasion of the virus. The tests for HIV search for these antibodies. It takes people anywhere from six weeks to six months for these antibodies to show up on the test. A person can be infected with HIV and still test negative when using the ELISA and the Western Blot tests if their body has not yet created the antibodies.

Children are born with the mother's antibodies so if the mother is HIV-positive, the child will be born positive. It can take up to 18 months for the child to seroconvert to negative if the child was not infected by the mother. Without treatment usually one out of three children born to an HIV-positive mother will not seroconvert, and will remain HIV-positive.

Seroconversion illness—when a person is first infected, within days or weeks they usually experience severe flu-like symptoms and/or have very swollen lymph glands.

STD's—sexually transmitted diseases such as gonorrhea, syphilis, clamidia, and genital warts, as well as HIV.

T-cell count—is a surrogate marker that is used to gauge progression of HIV. A healthy T-cell count is 500 to 1500. When your T-cells go under 200 you technically have AIDS, according to the CDC.

T-Cells—are white blood cells that help direct the body's infection-fighting cells. Also called CD4 cells and T helper cells.

3TC—is a reverse transcriptase inhibitor similar to AZT. Also known as Epivir and lamivudine.

Viral Load—is a surrogate marker that gauges the progression of HIV. This test actually measures the amount of virus in the peripheral blood (not in the lymph or any other organs). There are a number of different tests—under 5,000 copies/ml is thought to be okay, though many believe that it is best to achieve an undetectable viral load.

Western Blot Test—is a more precise test for the HIV antibodies. If you have been given the ELISA test and it comes back positive, they will give you the Western Blot test to confirm the diagnosis. They give the ELISA test first because it is less expensive.

Window Period—the period of time between when a person has been exposed to HIV and when they have created antibodies that would give them a positive result from taking either the ELISA test or the Western Blot test. It can range from six weeks to a year depending on the individual's immune system. The healthier the person, the quicker it will develop the antibodies.

Zovirax—prophylaxis that helps prevent herpes.

answers to common questions

What is the difference between HIV and AIDS?

Human immunodeficiency virus (HIV) is a virus that attacks infection-fighting blood cells and other parts of the immune system and is thought to cause AIDS. Acquired immunodeficiency syndrome is a collection of illnesses that a person becomes at risk for once the HIV has sufficiently destroyed the person's immune system. That is the physical differences. Culturally AIDS has been associated with a terminal condition, amounting to a virtual death sentence. In reality people go in and out of what constitutes an AIDS diagnosis. In other words they acquire opportunistic infections and then can heal from them. Subsequently a person diagnosed with AIDS can in fact live symptom-free for long periods of time. So when you feel that itch to ask the eternal question—'Do you have HIV or AIDS?'—stop yourself right there and know it is irrelevant. A person with *only* HIV can be at times sicker than someone diagnosed with AIDS. The diagnostic criteria is arbitrary. Being *just* HIV-positive does not make having this illness any easier.

Once the virus successfully destroys a part of a person's immune system that person can no longer fight infections that would normally not be a problem. He or she may also get life-threatening illnesses that a person with an a intact immune system might be able to survive, but because the immune system is compromised that person cannot fight the illness or tolerate the often toxic treatment. People don't die of AIDS, they die from the diseases that they can't fight because the HIV has destroyed their immune system. It is a long, slow, painful death.

Is the CDC being completely honest about nonsexual transmission?

I don't think they are trying to hide anything on purpose. They are certain how HIV is transmitted because they have tracked it through different people's behaviors at least in the beginning. People are concerned sometimes that it may be transmitted through other means than the ways disclosed by the CDC. If this were so then we would have a much greater degree of infection than we do. The cases where HIV was transmitted by obscure means are always media feasts and every one jumps on the story, such as with Kimberly Bergalis and the transmission from her dentist. That particular event was shrouded in mystery. Did he intentionally infect her and how?

We will never know. There have been other rare cases of transmission: e.g., sharing a toothbrush or a razor. There are precautions you should take when living with someone who is HIV and/or, for that matter, if they are not HIV. It is best not to share any implements that might have blood, semen, vaginal secretion or breast milk on them in a way that it might enter your bloodstream. I have to stress that even those incidents are rare and can be classified as 'freak' transmissions. As far as getting it by sitting next to someone or sharing the same soft drink, that has been proven to be impossible.

How can we prevent ourselves from becoming infected with HIV?

You might expect me to say 'Well that's obvious, don't let semen, vaginal secretions, blood, or breast milk enter your bloodstream through the rectum, vagina, mouth, or open wound'—but I feel it is more complicated than that. The behavior is often a symptom of what is going on at a deeper level. (It is important first and foremost to understand that.) Then it is important to put away whatever denial mechanisms you might incorporate to put a distance between you and the possibility of infection. HIV infection is real and it is in our communities. As you have seen on these pages it can infect anyone. Also we often engage in many unsafe behaviors out of pain, to kill the feelings that we are not good enough. I was

infected with HIV somewhere between 19 and 24, this was when I was at the lowest emotional point in my life. Now at 37 I am living with the consequences of my actions. I am not talking about punishment—just cause and effect. My life has changed drastically since then. I want to live. I would have a wonderful life if it wasn't for HIV. If I had known there was a contagious disease that would utterly change my life—at times making it unbearable—I never would have left myself vulnerable to contracting it.

I hope that all of you can see beyond your actions in the present day and reduce the risk of becoming infected by not allowing semen, vaginal secretion, blood, or breast milk to enter your blood stream. I know I said this twice before, but the terms 'unsafe behavior', 'abstinence', and 'safe sex' are just not specific enough. Become educated, learn about how to have satisfying safe sex or how to say no. There are many tragedies in life. Most of them are not preventable—HIV infection is. I would trade anything I have or have had to be free from AIDS.